COWBOYS AND INDIAN
THE GREAT BRITISH HOSPITAL OF TEXAS

SANDIP MATHUR, M.D.

© 2020, Sandip V. Mathur, M.D.

Genre: Creative Non-fiction

ISBN: 978-0-9973706-6-9

Designed by Tinyah M. Hawkins/Goofidity Designs

Cover photograph by Michelle Hanna

Printed in the USA

Published by TexasStarTrading.com
174 Cypress Street
Abilene, Texas 79601
info.TexasStar@yahoo.com
(325) 672-9696

To my wife and my family.
In memory of my father.

TABLE OF CONTENTS

Preface		1
Chapter 1	Man on Fire	3
Chapter 2	Now Meet the Family	18
Chapter 3	The Foreign Body	30
Chapter 4	The Friday Night Storm	46
Chapter 5	Love Thy Neighbor	57
Chapter 6	Horse Thieves Gulch	70
Chapter 7	Rodeo Drive	84
Chapter 8	The Board Meeting	103
Chapter 9	The Last Home Visit	116
Chapter 10	The Knife of the Party	127
Chapter 11	The Great British Hospital of Texas	146
Chapter 12	The Gifts of Christmas	154
Chapter 13	The Cattlewomen's Ball	175
Chapter 14	A Bad Stroke	184
Chapter 15	Measure for Measure	198
Chapter 16	Burned	214
Chapter 17	Awesome Dell Clawsom	240
Chapter 18	Strategy	270
Chapter 19	The Green Card Interview	289
Chapter 20	The King Returns	306
Chapter 21	Graveside Services	319

PREFACE

I finished my training in internal medicine and gastroenterology in 1995. I was married, with daughters two and five, and on a student visa. I was offered a job in rural West Texas. The county hospital was unable to recruit local doctors and offered us green cards if I practiced there for three years.

After London and Houston, living in a town of five thousand and working in an underserved hospital required a lot of adjustment. There were no other specialists and the lab and X-ray facilities were rudimentary. I relied on taking a detailed history, examining patients carefully, ordering the few tests available, and hunting for clues. I became a medical detective.

As an immigrant family, it was an adventure for all of us. We grappled with American customs, passions, and idiosyncrasies. The political correctness of big cities is absent in small towns; the American identity lies bare. We accepted the simple honesty and scrutiny of our new friends and carved out a life together.

These events happened over twenty years ago. I have tried to recreate events, locales, and conversations from my memory of them. In order to maintain their anonymity, I have changed the names of individuals, including my family, and places. I have also changed some identifying characteristics and details such as physical appearances, occupations, and places of residence. In my first book, *Cowboys and Indian: A Doctor's First Year in Texas*, I wrote an account of my introduction to West Texas. This book continues the narrative and covers the second year.

Many days were joyful, others heartbreaking; some bewildering and others hilarious, but *never* were they dull. That's the thrill of practicing medicine.

As an immigrant Indian family in the Bible belt, this was

an extraordinary experience for all of us. My contract stipulated that I stay there three years; we ended up spending six years instead. Through my writing, I hope I convey the friendship, love, and respect that emerged on both sides.

Sandip V. Mathur, M.D.

CHAPTER 1
MAN ON FIRE

We were in the Hotspur Hospital Emergency Room, just before midnight. There were two other medical personnel: Dr. Ehrlich and the ER nurse, Simon Godwyn.

Our patient, Guillermo Bolivar Gutierrez, was a sixty-four-year-old truck mechanic who had collapsed at home. He had stopped breathing by the time the ambulance arrived. They started chest compressions and got an IV going, and rushed him to our hospital.

Guillermo was over six feet and weighed at least three hundred pounds. He was strapped to the gurney, naked except for a blanket draped over his groin, twin IV lines in each forearm, and heart monitor leads that kept falling off his hairy chest. He jerked his arms and legs and twisted spasmodically. He coughed and retched repeatedly. The room reeked of diesel and vomit. The floor was littered with needle covers, blood-stained gauze, scraps of tape, EKG strips, plastic wrapping, IV cannulas, and chest electrodes. A pile of dirty towels, used to wipe the vomit, accumulated under the sink.

I stood above his head, wrenched his jaw up with one hand and crushed a plastic oxygen face mask over his nose and mouth with the other. Simon was on our patient's left side, performing chest compressions, and Dr. Ehrlich darted from the monitor to the patient.

Guillermo struggled, but was unable to move air. His chest rose slightly with each effort and collapsed quickly; his breathing had become infrequent. His sweaty face and body became turgid and went from blue to purple; his engorged veins stood out like ropes; his bloodshot eyes popped and careened wildly. He suddenly lunged towards Simon and retched. Simon jumped. Guillermo hacked and thrashed his legs. The gurney shuddered and Dr. Ehrlich held down Guillermo's feet. Simon arched over Guillermo again and resumed chest compressions, creating a trickle of circulation. We had been working for thirty minutes and we were exhausted. Dr. Ehrlich examined the rhythm on the heart monitor forlornly.

"Is there *any* bloody chance?" Simon gasped. He paused chest compressions and looked at me.

I squeezed the purple Ambu bag twice and thrust oxygen into Guillermo's lungs. His chest rose an inch, paused, and fell.

"I don't know," I answered. "We don't know how long he was down at home. At least he's moving some oxygen now, that's good."

"Continue compressions?" Simon asked.

"Yes! Keep up the compressions!" I ordered.

"*I'm* in charge here, not Dr. Mathur," Dr. Ehrlich snapped. "You take orders from *me!*"

"Yes, sir," Simon said.

"You two have got some kind of British connection going, I see that!" Dr. Ehrlich said. "You know what? I've been moonlighting in ERs for years, so I don't care. *I'm* in charge here!"

"Then what would *you* like me to do, *sir?*" Simon asked, sarcastically.

"Continue the compressions!" Dr. Ehrlich ordered.

Simon smirked and resumed the compressions. Guillermo's arms and head jerked with the compressions.

"*One*, two, three, four, five, six, *seven*," Simon grunted.

I looked at the cardiac monitor. The monitor showed large irregular waves.

"*Eight*, nine, ten, eleven," Simon glared at me.

"Doesn't look too good," I said.

"Hopeless!" Simon grunted.

I looked at the monitor and at Dr. Ehrlich. He looked away.

"Twelve, thirteen, fourteen, *fifteen!*" Simon announced, and straightened up abruptly.

I squeezed the oxygen bag twice. The man's chest rose and fell twice, but his face grew more bloated.

"We've been working on him for thirty minutes, sir," Simon protested.

"Hold compressions for ten seconds!" Dr. Ehrlich ordered abruptly. "Hold it! Hold it!"

Simon paused briefly; as we watched, the heart waves became very small and irregular. The oxygen level plummeted below sixty percent.

Simon shook his head wearily and resumed compressions. Guillermo's head bobbed and his limbs jerked.

"This is bonkers, Dr. Mathur!" Simon complained, and looked at me.   Dr. Ehrlich was furious.

"Why are you looking at him?" Dr. Ehrlich grabbed Simon's shoulder. "*I'm* running this code, *not* Dr. Mathur."

Simon glared at him.

"You want me to still keep going?" he asked, curtly.

"Did I tell you to stop?" Dr. Ehrlich asked. "Did you hear me say, Simon, stop?"

Simon shrugged.

"*Don't* stop the compressions! Keep going! Keep going!" Dr. Ehrlich ordered.

"Dr. Ehrlich, his oxygen level is low," I said. "He has a history of sleep apnea and he's a big boy. I'm having a hard time keeping his oxygen up."

"So what should we do about it, genius?"

"I think he needs a tube in his airway."

Dr. Ehrlich hesitated.

"You *think*?" he sneered.

"I am *sure* we need an airway. I can do it," I replied, irritated. I brandished an endotracheal tube.

Dr. Ehrlich snorted and stepped back.

"No. Too risky," he said. "Put it away."

"His oxygen level is 88 percent, even though we're blasting him with 100 percent oxygen. That's not good."

"I know that's not good! Don't try to teach me medicine!"

"So should I intubate?" I persisted.

"No, too risky."

"Even more risky to leave him without an airway."

Dr. Ehrlich came up to me and grabbed my forearm.

"*I'm* running this code! I'm telling you, no intubation!"

"Okay, no intubation," I said. I shook him off. But I slipped the endotracheal tube under Guillermo's neck, just in case.

Dr. Ehrlich glared at the patient.

"These arm IVs are so damn useless!" he complained. He whipped the towel off and cleaned the right groin with alcohol.

"They put the IVs in the elbows!" he went on. "Which idiot did that? Every time he bends his arms they block off!"

"That's the best I could get," Simon admitted.

"Is that what they taught you in London? Start IVs in the worst possible places?" Dr. Ehrlich taunted.

He swabbed the groin with alcohol-soaked gauze and cleaned it off with iodine. He covered the genitalia with the towel and pushed them away from the thigh. He palpated the femoral artery with the fingertips of his left hand and, with his right, inserted a thick needle a quarter-inch vertically into the tissue a half-inch away from the artery. He pulled back on the syringe. Dark red blood welled up for an instant and stopped. He poked again and pulled back. No more blood came back.

"Try a little closer to the artery, angulate," I suggested.

Dr. Ehrlich grunted. He started again, a little closer, and inserted the needle at a forty-five degree angle. He drew back and suctioned. Nothing. He glared at me.

"You have to go closer to the artery," I said. "Go closer and deeper. He's a big boy!"

"Shut up! I don't need your advice, damn it!" Dr. Ehrlich shouted, and did exactly as I advised.

There was a spurt of crimson.

"I'm in!" he whooped. "Give me the damn guide wire!"

Simon nudged the set, taking care not to touch the sterile contents. Dr. Ehrlich pulled out a long thin wire. His success softened him.

"I know it looks bad," he admitted, and threaded the wire through the thick needle, "but at least we now have good IV access. Not those damn useless IVs in the elbows!"

He glared at Simon and removed the needle and slid a plastic catheter over the guide wire.

"Hold compressions!" he ordered, and swiftly stitched the catheter to the skin. He connected it to the bag of saline and checked.

"*Now* it's flowing! Good!" he said. He covered Guillermo's groin with Tegaderm, sterile cling-film, to seal the area.

"Good job, Doc," Simon muttered sarcastically. "You saved him where all of us failed!"

Dr. Ehrlich ignored Simon's needling.

"What are you waiting for? Resume compressions!" he ordered.

"We can send that blood for electrolytes," I suggested.

"I *know* what to do! I don't need your expert advice for anything, genius!" Dr. Ehrlich said. He squirted the blood into red, blue and pink-topped tubes. He hesitated.

"Um, what's the number for your lab?" he asked, quietly.

Tom, the chief lab tech, was there in seconds. He was a tall, lean man with thick white hair, brushed neatly. He checked the tubes.

"You want me to run some arterial blood gases as well?" he asked.

I smiled. Tom was experienced.

"Oh! Yes! Yes!" Dr. Ehrlich stammered. "I was *just* about to do that! Just about to get some arterial blood!"

"I'll start running these and come back. I guess you need electrolytes and hemoglobin stat?" Tom said, smoothly.

"Yes," Dr. Ehrlich drew up a bead of heparin in a five cc syringe.

"Calcium and magnesium?" Tom asked.

Dr. Ehrlich squirmed.

"Yes, yes, *yes!*"

Tom disappeared.

Dr. Ehrlich stabbed the left femoral artery and slowly withdrew the needle. Nothing.

"His blood pressure is low, so it's difficult to get the artery," he declared.

He swabbed the groin again. He shifted and thrust the needle in at a different angle. He withdrew cautiously.

Nothing.

"Damn!" he exclaimed. He changed his angle and thrust the needle again. A jet of crimson shot up.

Guillermo suddenly drew his legs up and cried out. He knocked Dr. Ehrlich to the floor. The syringe and needle burst out of his hands, sailed in an arc, and fell into the sink.

"I guess you *did* get his artery!" Simon smirked.

"Restrain him! *Restrain him!*" Dr. Ehrlich cried, scrambling up.

Guillermo retched and threw up again. Thick green liquid burst out, covered his face and chest, and sprayed my hands and Simon's shirt and neck. The stench flooded the room. We wiped Guillermo's face and chest and suctioned food out of his mouth.

I turned angrily to Dr. Ehrlich.

"I need to put in an airway!" I repeated. "We have to protect his lungs! We don't want him sucking stomach contents into his lungs!"

Dr. Ehrlich froze.

Simon wiped his arms and face. There was mutiny everywhere.

"I'm tired, sir," Simon declared.

"I'll take over," I said and moved to the side. Simon moved to the head and grasped the bag.

Dr. Ehrlich shuddered. He glared at Simon.

"Too weak to do compressions, eh? Okay. Bag him. One squeeze every fifteen compressions!" Dr. Ehrlich reminded him, scornfully.

"You don't have to tell me, I know," Simon said. "They *did* teach us that in London."

Dr. Ehrlich stared at him with disgust.

"It's been almost thirty-six minutes now," I announced.

"Thank you!" Dr. Ehrlich hissed. "You have an amazing grasp of the obvious!"

I completed another fifteen compressions and spoke.

"He may be low in potassium. Look at the EKG. The complexes are pretty small," I said.

Dr. Ehrlich threw his arms up.

"Potassium! Where are the labs? We need the potassium level! Damn! Freaking useless ER!" Dr. Ehrlich wailed. "Can't even get a lousy chemistry report!"

"Call the lab and ask Tom," Simon suggested. "Extension two-two-four."

"*You* call them," Dr. Ehrlich ordered, and took over the oxygen bag from Simon. I continued compressions.

"Why do I have to push so hard with the bag?" Dr. Ehrlich complained. "There's too much resistance!"

"That's what I said," I countered. "I told you there was a lot of airway resistance and that I should intubate."

"I didn't know it was *this* much resistance! This is too much! I'm having to really work to get oxygen into him!"

"So should I intubate?" I asked.

Dr. Ehrlich hesitated.

"You think you can get it? He's a big man."

"I think so. If you or Simon help me, I can do it."

I grabbed the intubation cart. Dr. Ehrlich squeezed the bag four times to give Guillermo a boost of oxygen.

Simon looked up from the phone.

"Potassium is three-point-one, sir," he announced. "Normal is three-point-five to five-point-two."

I looked at the EKG recordings on the monitor.

"Dr. Ehrlich, I still think the EKG complexes are too small; that happens when the blood potassium is too low."

"No, I don't think so, genius," Dr. Ehrlich countered. "He's just fat."

"Look how small the complexes are and how slow the heart rate is," I pointed out.

"Doesn't prove anything!"

"He's on Lasix, lots of Lasix, and that pulls potassium out of the body, and he recently took Zaroxylin," I said.

"So what? His potassium is low but not *very* low."

"You struggled so much to get his blood!" I said.

"I got the central line in his femoral!" Dr. Ehrlich said proudly.

"Yes, but you had to try repeatedly, and that hemolyzes and

damages the red cells, they leak potassium, and that *raises* the blood potassium level. The normal potassium is three-point-five in our lab so three-point-one is low and it's really probably *even* lower, given that there's hemolysis," I said, between compressions.

"No hemolysis! Forget the potassium! Just intubate him, genius!"

Dr. Ehrlich took over compressions. I squeezed the bag repeatedly, flooding the lungs with plenty of oxygen. He would be without any oxygen until I got a tube into his airway.

If I got a tube into his airway.

I strapped on a face mask. I slid my thumb inside his mouth and pulled up on his chin. I forced his mouth wide open. He moved from side to side, and suddenly coughed forcefully. A spray of grey sticky sputum coated my face mask.

"Suction! Give me suction!" I demanded. I wiped my mask clean on the side of the bed.

Dr. Ehrlich swung around and grabbed the suction catheter.

"I knew you couldn't do it!" he said, victoriously.

I suctioned the oral cavity. The back of his mouth was obscured by two enormous tonsils and his fleshy soft palate hung down over them like a shroud. I couldn't see the larynx.

I threw off the face mask. No better.

"You won't be able to do it!" Dr. Ehrlich predicted, happily.

"I can't see the airway!" I admitted.

"I knew it! I told you it wouldn't work!" Dr. Ehrlich trilled.

"I'm going to try with the tongue blade. Give me a medium Mackintosh!"

Simon snatched a Mackintosh tongue blade and snapped it onto a handle. I grabbed it without looking away.

"Suction him!" I ordered.

I slipped in the tongue blade and hooked it around the back of the tongue and pulled up. I got a brief glimpse of a tube with white tissue.

"I think I see the cords!"

"You *think?*" Dr. Ehrlich scoffed.

I tugged harder.

"Yes! I see them! Give me an eight ET tube!"

Simon squirted lubricating jelly on an endotracheal tube and slammed a metal stiffener into it. I grabbed it.

I saw the larynx bob in and out of view.

"Hold the compressions!" I shouted.

I pulled harder on the jaw and saw the larynx again. I thrust the plastic tube in like a spear.

There was an awful moment of silence.

Then Guillermo's chest deflated two inches. The plastic tube steamed over with the moisture of the released air.

"I think I'm in!" I whooped.

I inflated the balloon that secured the tube and connected it to the oxygen bag. I squeezed mightily, not daring to breathe.

Guillermo's chest rose and sank. Water vapor streaked the tubing.

"Yes! I'm in! Listen for lung sounds!"

Dr. Ehrlich listened to both sides of the chest, then nodded reluctantly.

"You're in," he said drily. "Wonderful."

A plump, middle-aged woman burst into the room, clutching a baby and dragging a young girl, probably ten. They were panic-stricken.

"*Es mi esposo!* My husband!" she cried.

Dr. Ehrlich quickly placed an arm around her shoulder and wheeled her around. The ten-year-old stared wide-eyed at her father.

"We are doing everything we can," Dr. Ehrlich said softly. "I want you to wait outside."

"No, no, I want to stay here, with my husband," she wailed. She struggled to get free. Her daughter began to hiccup.

Dr. Ehrlich did not relent. He grasped the daughter's shoulder and dragged them to the door.

"We are doing *everything* possible, we are doing *everything*. Just wait outside here, and let us do our job," he said firmly.

"Is he going to *die?*" she asked, her pitch rising. "Is he going to *die?*"

"We are doing everything," Dr. Ehrlich repeated, and held up his hands. His wife's face cracked in horror. The daughter started shaking.

"O Dio mio, he *is* going to die!" she wailed. "Dio mio, Dio mio!"

"No, no, he is *not* going to die! Just stay out here and wait!"

Dr. Ehrlich put both arms around her and guided her through the door.

"You too!" he said to the ten year old. She swayed and obeyed.

"But I want to be with my husband!" the wife protested.

"Let us do our job, ma'am," Dr. Ehrlich insisted. "Wait here, I will come back to you as soon as I can."

She lunged back past Dr. Ehrlich and grasped her husband's ankle.

"I want to stay!" she repeated. "Let me stay!"

Dr. Ehrlich peeled her hand away.

"No!" he shouted. "No! Now go!"

"Let me stay!"

"No! Did you not hear me? I said no!"

He pushed them into the corridor and slammed the door hard. It hit the frame, shuddered, and swung open again, revealing the astonished wife and daughter.

Dr. Ehrlich closed the door again with cautious majesty and jammed a stool against it.

"Does *nothing* work in this useless ER?" he spat, "not even the *doors* close?"

The door creaked a little. He ignored it.

"How many minutes has it been?" he asked.

"Almost forty-eight minutes," Simon replied.

"I still think we need to give him potassium," I repeated.

"You have said that many times, Dr. Mathur, and I have said no. I know you trained in some very fancy hospitals in London and Houston. But *I'm* in charge here. The blood potassium level is good enough!"

"So what should we do?" I asked, irritated.

"Change the chest leads! He's a big hairy man and the hair and fat is why he has small waves!" Dr. Ehrlich said.

"Should I replace the leads or reposition? Or do *anything* you recommend?" Simon asked, his voice dripping with bitterness.

Dr. Ehrlich turned red.

"Just fix it!" he screamed. "Fix the damn leads!"

Simon replaced the leads and we scanned the monitor again. Small, rapid waves.

"Blood pressure?" Dr Ehrlich asked.

"Fifty systolic," I answered.

"Not good enough!"

"How about trying some potassium?" I asked.

"No! It's the leads!"

"Should I shave his chest?" Simon asked. "Better contact for the leads, what?"

"Waste of time! He needs to be shocked. I'm going to shock him," Dr. Ehrlich announced.

"Simon, I'm tired. Take over compressions," I ordered. "Give me the bag."

We exchanged positions.

"What kind of outdated cardiac defibrillator is this?" Dr.

Ehrlich complained, dragging the cart closer to the patient.

"It's an old model, but it's pretty good. Set it to 'synchronised shock' and dial it up to three hundred volts," I said.

"I know that, genius doctor, thank you," Dr. Ehrlich muttered, and obeyed.

"I think you will need to shave his chest quickly, he's got a very hairy chest," I pointed out.

Dr. Ehrlich looked at me angrily.

"Am I blind? Am I blind? Do you think I am blind? You think I can't see that?"

"No, I just want to tell you to shave the chest quickly."

"Did I *ask* for your opinion?" he hissed. "Did I?"

He pulled the paddles off the defibrillator. He looked at the controls.

"How do I get it to three hundred joules?" he asked, quietly.

"There's a dial on the right side," Simon pointed out. "Turn it clockwise."

Dr. Ehrlich dialed three hundred. The defibrillator hummed loudly, then gave three beeps and flashed 300 in green over the EKG.

"It's ready," Simon declared.

"Stand back!" Dr. Ehrlich ordered.

Simon and I stepped back.

Dr. Ehrlich applied the paddles to the chest and squeezed the buttons viciously.

There was a *whump* and Gilberto's body jerked. We watched the monitor.

"No change!" Dr. Ehrlich declared. "Go up to three hundred sixty joules!"

"Just dial it up again, sir," Simon instructed. "Same way."

Dr. Ehrlich repeated the exercise. The room smelled of burnt hair.

"At least put something on his chest to improve the contact of the paddles," I said.

"Where are the contact gel pads?" Dr. Ehrlich demanded.

"We don't have them, we just use alcohol wipes to swab the chest," Simon said.

"No gel pads? I give up!" Dr Ehrlich said angrily. "What kind of an ER is this?"

Simon reached over and gave him a box of alcohol wipes.

"A poor one. A poor ER. Welcome to the real world," he said.

Dr. Ehrlich tossed the box aside.

"Have you seen his chest? How hairy! He needs a lot of alcohol, not just a few useless swabs!"

He grabbed a bottle of methyl alcohol and splashed it on the patient's chest. He soaked a piece of gauze in alcohol and spread it all around.

He turned back and dialed the defibrillator to three hundred and sixty. It hummed loudly and beeped again.

"Stand back! Stand back! Three hundred and sixty joules!" he warned.

We stood back again.

Dr. Ehrlich hesitated. He rested one paddle on the patient's sternum and looked for a place to rest the other. His hands trembled. The defibrillator gave a warning signal.

"You've got to shock him now," Simon warned, "or it will switch off!"

Dr. Ehrlich froze.

"Now! *Now!*" Simon hollered.

Suddenly there was a blue flash over the patient's chest. Small flames danced on Guillermo's chest. The odor of burnt skin and hair burst like a grenade.

"He's on fire!" Simon cried out in horror.

There were low blue flames flickering on Guillermo's chest!

I lunged forward and grabbed the towel covering his groin and pounded the chest furiously. Dr. Ehrlich remained frozen, his mouth open, with the paddles in mid-air.

"What just happened?" Simon asked aloud.

Dr. Ehrlich quickly replaced the paddles and was silent.

"What just happened?" Simon demanded again, loudly.

"What's the rhythm?" I asked.

There was no rhythm at all. There was only a flat line.

"Do *something!*" I begged Dr. Ehrlich.

He remained frozen.

I turned to Simon.

"Give him potassium!" I yelled. "*Potassium!* Forty of potassium!"

"*No!*" Dr. Ehrlich screamed.

"Give it!" I ordered, yelling louder.

Simon snatched up a vial of potassium and drew it up in a sixty cc syringe. Dr. Ehrlich grabbed his wrist.

"If you give it, you're fired!" he threatened.

I snatched the syringe and needle from Simon and rammed it into a hub on the tubing.

"Don't you *dare* give it!" Dr. Ehrlich warned, his face seething.

I injected it very slowly, watching the rhythm.

It remained flat. We waited another minute in silence.

Still flat.

Another minute.

Flat line for four minutes.

Dr. Ehrlich screamed and turned to me, his voice shaking with fury.

"You gave him potassium! You killed him! You're *fired!*"

CHAPTER 2
NOW MEET THE FAMILY

Twelve hours later, I entered David Dawkins' office. David was the hospital administrator. He was about five feet ten, plump, bald, and sported half-moon glasses. He looked upset. He threw down a file and pushed back from his desk. He waved me in.

"Good Lord, Doc!" he said. "You really are in deep trouble!"

"I know," I said. "How bad is it?"

I walked through the green shag carpet and perched at the edge of the yellow chair facing him. I knew not to sit back in it.

David shook his head. He looked at me above his glasses.

"Real bad. You sure pissed him off, Doc!" he said. "Doc Ehrlich says you killed the patient! He's written to the State Board in Austin and the Hospital Board!"

"I can explain."

David tossed his glasses on his desk.

"Oh, you *definitely* have to explain. You'll have to explain to the Hospital Board, explain to the State Board, but most of all, you'll have to explain to the family why you set him on fire, then gave him a wallop of potassium, and hope they won't sue the pants off you and the hospital."

"I didn't set him on fire, Dr. Ehrlich did. I pushed some potassium because I thought his blood level was low. It was a last-ditch effort, the man was almost dead. I had to do something! Really, I can explain."

David shook his head.

"What's this about the State Board?" I asked.

"You'll have to explain to the State Board about the potassium, and pray they don't pull your license."

"What do you mean?"

"Dr. Ehrlich said that you pushed potassium and that killed him."

"That's ridiculous. The potassium was already low on the blood test, and I was sure it was actually even lower. Like I said, I gave some potassium as a last-ditch effort to save the patient."

"Your buddy, Dr. Ehrlich, sent a formal complaint to the Hospital Board and to Austin, and asked for an inquiry about the potassium you pushed."

"That's crazy! I'm sure I'm right about the potassium. And *he* was the one who set the patient on fire!"

"Well, he wasn't clear about that. But he did say that you pushed potassium against his advice, and the patient died."

"The patient had already flat-lined! I tried to save him!" I protested.

David waved.

"Right now, we got a bereaved family outside, wanting to know why their daddy is dead."

I stood up.

"Then let Ehrlich come and tell them. He was the one in charge, as he said a hundred times."

"He's gone back to Dallas," David said.

"I thought he was covering the whole week of Thanksgiving," I said.

"We couldn't afford it. You know the hospital is pretty tight. Your immigration lawyer costs a hundred twenty-five an hour! So no coverage till Friday night. Ehrlich's coming back for the weekend."

"So I'm on call till the weekend?"

"Yes."

I had not expected that.

"Hey, you're alone at home. Your wife and kids have gone to

Canada," David went on casually, "so I figured, you got nothing to do, so you can take call."

"How did you know about Maya and the girls?" I asked.

David grinned.

"Small town, Doc. Everyone knows everything," he explained.

I was irritated.

"I only came in to help last night. I wasn't even on call."

"No good deed goes unpunished. Doc. Ehrlich called you in?"

"No, the nurse, Simon."

"That British nurse? Two foreigners against a good old boy? Not good, not good. You're up a creek without a paddle, Doc!"

I didn't know what to say.

David leaned forward and lowered his voice.

"I got to ask this favor," he said softly.

"What's that?"

"Talk to the family real nice. Calm them down. Help them understand and forgive whatever the hell happened. Tell them Ehrlich did his best," David pleaded.

"Are you *kidding?*" I exploded. "Are you crazy? Ehrlich complained about me to the board, and I should *defend* him?"

"Doc, right now, we got a bereaved family. Just lost their dad, husband, whatever. They're going to be emotional. Just calm them down, explain what happened."

"Why are you defending Ehrlich?"

"I'm defending the hospital. We can't afford a lawsuit. I don't want them suing us."

"Then call Ehrlich. He was in charge."

"He's not here, I told you. Forget about the potassium deal, for now."

"The patient was flat-lining! I had to do *something!*" I raged.

"You had to do something? The man's almost dead, and *then* you jump in?" David shook his head in disbelief.

"He wasn't dead, he was dying! I was sure his potassium was low!"

"According to Dr. Ehrlich, the potassium was three-point-two. Low, but not that low," David countered.

"Look, David, the normal potassium is three point five to five in our lab. It has to be within that narrow range, otherwise heart medicines don't work," I explained.

"The potassium was not *seriously* low," David repeated, unmoved.

I leaned in and kept my voice calm.

"Listen to me. Dr. Ehrlich had a hard time drawing that sample. That crushed the red blood cells and released potassium."

"So what?"

"So that reported not-so-low value of three point two in that sample was actually artificially *higher* than the true value," I explained. "The *real* potassium in the blood must have been much lower. Probably below three, maybe two point nine."

"So when you draw a blood sample the potassium always goes up?" David asked, confused.

"No, only when the sample isn't obtained smoothly. If you poke several times and pull hard to get blood, that crushes the red blood cells and releases potassium because they have lots of potassium inside them."

David stared at me and shook his head. He toyed with a pencil.

"Anything else you want to say?" he demanded, jabbing the pencil at me.

"I saw Dr. Ehrlich obtain the sample. He struggled. Simon can back me up. And the patient was on Zaroxylin. That's a very powerful diuretic. It makes the kidneys lose lots of potassium."

David sighed and looked out the window. He studied the old grey lamp posts outside and fell silent.

"I understand," he said eventually.

But he didn't turn back. He avoided looking at me.

"So where do we stand?" I asked.

"You're still in deep trouble, Doc," he said. "You haven't got your green card yet. And the hospital is also in deep trouble financially. We can barely afford your immigration lawyer. We just can't afford a lawsuit. It'll kill us."

"What do I do?"

David turned and folded his hands.

"Talk to the family. Please! Explain nicely, calmly. Widow and brother are here and the sister-in-law is coming later," David said.

"There's a lot of people waiting outside," I replied. "I just saw them. Big family."

"Already?" David turned pale.

"Yes, they're all waiting outside."

"That's the Hispanic panic. They all show up in force when something happens," David said ruefully.

David snatched a card off his desk and scurried to the door.

"Hope you're ready for this!" he called out.

He disappeared into the secretary's office. I heard the other door open.

David coughed loudly and announced.

"Mr. Army Joe?"

There was silence.

"Mr. Army Joe?"

Silence.

"Um, okay. Mrs. Gutierrez?"

There was a murmur. Seconds later, he ushered the brother and wife into the room. I stood up and shook hands with the brother.

He was a thinner, shorter version of Guillermo. He had curly black hair, bright black eyes, and was clean-shaven. He wore a dark suit but no tie. Guillermo's wife, Adriana, wore a dark green sweatshirt and jeans. Her face was red and swollen, and she wiped her eyes repeatedly with her fingers.

"This is Dr. Mathur," David introduced. "He was there last night with Dr. Ehrlich."

Adriana nodded. We hugged. I shook hands with them.

"My name's pronounced Ar-mee-ho, not army-joe," the brother said, coldly. He handed me his card.

Armijo Bolivar Gutierrez PhD, University of Texas At Arlington, I read.

"I'm so sorry," David stammered.

"It happens," Armijo shrugged. "White people can't speak Spanish to save their lives."

"Sit down, sit down, please," David stammered.

There were only two yellow chairs for guests, so I remained standing. The brother and wife sat down and promptly sank. Mrs. Gutierrez remained prolapsed but Armijo grabbed the arms, pulled himself up, and perched on the edge. He glared at David. I stood near Adriana.

"I'm Dr. Mathur. I was one of the doctors looking after Mr. Guillermo last night. I'm very sorry about what happened," I said.

Mrs. Gutierrez sobbed. Armijo leaned over and squeezed her hand.

I pulled over a small filing cabinet and sat on it. David sat down in his chair.

"Guillermo was very ill," I started, cautiously.

"Guillermo! Ai, mi Guillermo!" his wife sobbed loudly. Armijo nodded slowly.

"Brother had chest pain for weeks and didn't want to see a doctor," he said.

"I begged him," his wife whispered hoarsely. "Begged him. No, he said, no, no, no."

"How long had this been going on?" I asked.

"Three or four weeks," she said. "He doubled all his heart medicines."

"Did he double the water pills?"

"He just said he doubled all his heart medicines," she repeated.

"I was worried that the potassium might have been too low, because water pills can pull off potassium as well as water. Did he take potassium pills?" I asked.

"Potassium? You mean those big pills?" she replied. "He had them but he didn't like to take them. They stick in his chest. So he stopped them."

I glanced at David.

"Those pills are notorious for being hard to swallow. Unfortunately, the potassium could have become very low," I explained.

I glanced at Armijo.

"Yes, I understand, Doctor," Armijo nodded.

"Potassium is very critical for the body," I explained. "Doubling the pill that takes water and potassium out of the body and not taking potassium replacements is dangerous."

Armijo coughed. There was an awkward silence.

"The family has a question. Did anything go wrong with the medical care last night?" he asked, quietly.

There was silence. I paused to think.

"Did anything go wrong with the care for my brother?" he repeated, sharply.

"Yes," I answered, "there was an accident. At one point,

there was too much alcohol on your brother's chest and a spark ignited it."

Armijo looked stunned.

"You *burned* him? You set him *on fire?* How could this happen?" Armijo burst out, furiously.

"Your brother had a very hairy chest. The leads kept falling off. We shaved as much as we could and then cleaned with alcohol. The spark came because the paddles were not touching the chest properly when the shock was given."

Armijo stared at me.

"Was it you?" he asked.

"No," I answered.

"Dr. Ehrlich?" Armijo asked.

"Yes," I admitted, "but it was an accident."

"Is that what killed him?"

"No, that didn't kill him. We put it out right away."

"Then what did kill him?" Armijo asked, angrily.

I thought for a minute.

"My opinion is that he had poor circulation in his heart, what we call unstable angina. He should have had a heart stent or bypass as soon as it began."

"Why didn't you send him for it last night?"

"By the time he came to us in the ER it was too late. He would have died on the way to Abilene. His heart went into a bad rhythm and stopped pumping properly. We tried and tried but we could not get him out of the bad rhythm," I explained.

"Why could you not get him out of the bad rhythm?" Armijo demanded. "*Why?* What happened?"

"We tried all the correct medicines and shocked him, we followed all the recommended protocols. I think he had lost so much potassium that the medicines did not work."

Armijo pondered briefly.

"The low potassium was caused by his taking too much medicine without supervision?" he asked.

"Yes," I replied.

"How low was the potassium?"

"Three point two."

"That's not *very* low," Armijo said sharply.

I was surprised.

"I think the real level was lower, because the blood sample was obtained with difficulty. That causes the red cells to get crushed and leak potassium so the levels seem to be higher than they really are," I explained.

Armijo stared at me, then nodded.

"I do understand. You had a hemolyzed sample. Makes sense," he turned to Adriana and nodded.

He chuckled at my surprise.

"I'm an assistant professor of biology at UT Arlington. Guillermo was my older brother. Our middle brother lives in San Antonio. Guillermo made me study for all of us," he explained.

"I'm sorry for your loss," I said. "I know that sounds hollow."

Armijo nodded. He looked at Adriana and nodded again.

"Okay. I read the ER notes already. I feel you did everything," he said.

He stood up abruptly and shook my hand.

"Now I understand why you gave that potassium," he said.

"I'm sure the potassium was lower than three," I explained.

"I agree, it was a reasonable choice."

"You agree?" David asked, surprised.

"Of course. You have someone on diuretics who doubles the dose and doesn't take his potassium, what do you expect?" Armijo said.

I was enormously relieved.

"I'm so glad you understand! I was worried," I admitted.

"Worried that we might sue you?" Armijo asked.

David laughed nervously and stood up to usher them out.

"Yes," I said.

Armijo shrugged.

"Yes, I thought about suing you. I thought about it a lot," he stated.

David wobbled and sat down again. Armijo looked at me and shook his head in sorrow.

"It was God's will. That's what I think now. I wasn't sure when we walked in, but your explanation makes me feel better. You did what you could. I wanted to hear you out."

Adriana looked up.

"I know you did everything you could. I watched from outside, the door wasn't closed," she said.

David looked at me.

"When Dr. Ear Lick set him *on fire*," she went on, "when he set him *on fire*, I knew you all had done everything, *everything* you could possibly do for him."

Armijo looked at her and shook his head. He turned to me, suddenly serious again.

"Explain to her why that happened," he said. "She didn't hear a word of what you said!"

I considered my words, then spoke slowly.

"Your husband had a hairy chest. The heart monitor leads kept falling off his chest. We put a lot of alcohol on him to improve the contact. When Dr. Ehrlich tried to give an electric shock to stimulate the heart, he was just a little bit off the skin and there was a spark. The spark made the hair burn."

"So it *was* a mistake?" she asked, sharply.

"Yes. It was a mistake," I said.

"Doctor, was this a *big* mistake?" she asked.

"What do you mean?"

"That's why he died?"

"No. But it didn't help."

"Made it worse?" Armijo asked.

"Yes, but it didn't cause his death."

"Was this a serious mistake on the part of Dr. Ehrlich?" Armijo persisted. "I mean, does this kind of thing just *happen?*"

I looked at David. He was watching me with concern.

"No," I said firmly, "but it was not a big mistake."

Armijo pressed the issue.

"Listen, doctor. We are not going to sue the hospital, okay? Just tell me, was that a serious mistake? Only someone like you, a doctor who has been in the same situation, knows the answer."

I looked at him.

"It was a mistake but not a serious mistake," I repeated.

Armijo looked straight at me.

"Could *you* have made that mistake?" Armijo asked.

"What do you mean?" I said, flustered.

"I know you are experienced, I read about you. So my question is, doctor, could *you* have made that mistake? Someone with your skills and experience? Could *you* have made that mistake and set my brother on fire?"

The prospect of nailing Dr. Ehrlich was appealing. A lawsuit for setting someone on fire! It would ravage him! I *could* get him sued. It was so tempting.

"Could *you* have made that mistake, Doctor?" Armijo repeated, speaking slowly and carefully.

I surprised myself with my response.

"Yes."

"Yes?" Armijo queried.

"Yes, I could have made that mistake."

"Really?" Armijo asked.

I nodded. It was the truth.

Armijo and I shook hands.

"Thank you, doctor," he said quietly.

Adriana pulled herself out of the chair and straightened up. She hugged me again.

"I believe you, Doctor," she said. "God bless you! God bless this little hospital!"

She hugged me again and they left. David slumped and covered his head with his hands.

CHAPTER 3

THE FOREIGN BODY

It rained all day Thanksgiving. I was watching the evening news when the phone rang.

"Dr. Mathur? It's Simon. I'm covering the ER tonight."

"Yes. I worked with you Sunday," I said.

"Yes, on Mr. Gutierrez. Pity about that," he said.

"Very sad. I spoke to the family afterwards," I said.

"How did they take it?"

"They were upset, naturally. They wanted to know what exactly had happened. I explained everything."

"Were they okay with it?" Simon wondered.

"I think so."

Simon paused.

"Well, I thought *you* did everything properly," he said.

"Thank you. By the way, that was the first time I met you. I wanted to welcome you to Hotspur. I assume you're British," I said.

"Yes, that's correct. From Coventry, actually, northwest of London. Betrothed to a local gal."

"I hope you enjoy Texas. Much more sunshine than London. I trained there for four years."

"Oh, did you? Which hospital?"

"Royal Hampstead Hospital in Belsize Park."

"Very nice! That's a famous teaching hospital."

"Yes. I had a good time there. You have a patient in the ER?"

"Yes, Dr. Mathur. It's a young man with a foreign body."

"Where is the foreign body?" I asked.

Simon coughed.

"Well, it's in his rectum, Dr. Mathur."

"In his *rectum?* What is it?"

Simon hesitated.

"It appears to be, based on the young man's description, the orange cap that previously resided on the top of a small can of shaving cream," he said.

"How did that get into his rectum?"

"He says he sat on it. By mistake."

I paused.

"He sat on it, by mistake," I repeated, "and he wasn't wearing any trousers or underwear?"

Simon ignored my sarcasm.

"There's a lady with him. His friend. She says she knows you. Her name's Patricia White."

"Yes, I do know her. What's she doing there?"

"She brought him in. He didn't know what to do."

"Is he bleeding?"

"Yes, and he is *very uncomfortable.*"

"I'll be right there."

"Oh, Dr. Mathur, I should warn you. It's been raining and the parking lot is a bloody swamp."

"I'll park on the road. Thanks."

I parked on the road and walked through the parking lot. It was still drizzling. There were two trucks parked by the ramp leading to the ER: a white Chevy, the sides thickly layered with mud, and a brown Toyota Tacoma, splattered front and sides. I glanced inside the Chevy. The cab was clean. There was a phone holder on the dash that was labeled *Argyris Garage*. The interior of the Toyota was a mess, with newspapers, batteries, shoes, cigarettes, a pair of long scissors, and pieces of stained cloth scattered about.

Simon was waiting for me in the corridor.

"Hello again, Dr. Mathur!" Simon said, holding out his hand.

We shook warmly. He was six feet, blond, clean-shaven, with sharp features and green eyes.

"Good evening. Pleasure," I said

"Simon Godwyn, RN, it's my pleasure entirely," he enthused. "Smashing to meet someone from England in this neck of the woods!"

"Brings back many happy memories of London. What have you got for me here, Simon?" I said.

"I wanted to catch you here in the corridor, Dr. Mathur. I wanted to tell you that this young man is rather upset."

"Upset? That he has a plastic cap in his rectum?"

"He is a young man and he's rather embarrassed, and Miss White is trying to add some levity to the situation, and he's not happy,"

"He's not happy with the situation or with Miss White?"

"Both, but mostly with Miss White," Simon explained.

"I understand. I know Miss White," I reassured him.

The ER in Hotspur was a small yellow rectangular box with a single small window on one long side and both doors on the other. One door opened to the corridor, and the other one, to the dictation cubicle. The examination light hung low. The walls were stained and blistered with chemical splashes, and several feet near the sink were bloated from water damage. Two resuscitation carts, two monitors, several IV poles and a half-dozen wheeled metal tables were crammed together, and glass cabinets with bags of saline and Ringer's lactate crowded the back wall. The dictation cubicle contained a rickety table and a red telephone.

The ER reeked of iodine and cigarette smoke.

Jerald Guthrie jumped when he saw me. He was about five nine, muscular, with matted blond hair in a mullet. He was drying his hair with a towel. He stood up, said nothing, and sat down again. His T-shirt said *Argyris Garage*.

I turned to his companion.

"Hello Tricia!" I said. "Long time no see!"

Tricia grinned and hugged me. She was thin, heavily tattooed, and had a smoker's cough.

"Sorry I didn't follow up," she said, hoarsely. "Couldn't afford it. But you fixed me up!"

"I'm glad you're better."

"Now I want you to help Jerry!" she declared.

Jerald stood up, flushed.

"This is Jerry," Tricia introduced, "Jerry, this is Dr. Sandy. I can't say his last name, but he's a good doc. He figured out I had a bacterial infection in my heart. Would have died if he hadn't fixed me!"

I remembered her presentation. She had been very ill.

"You look much better than last time!" I enthused. "So everything did work out? You got antibiotics for the full six weeks?"

"You bet! And they had medical students coming to look at my eyes all the time I was there!" she said.

I turned to Jerry.

"Hi! I'm Dr. Mathur."

Jerry shook hands cautiously.

"I saw you today," he said. "You were coming to my neighbors, the Parrishs, around noon. You had an umbrella and a bottle of wine."

"Yes, they had invited me for Thanksgiving lunch. I'm alone right now; my wife and kids are in Canada. So what happened, Jerry?"

Jerry looked at Tricia.

"You don't have to be scared, Jer!" Tricia said. "He's nice. *I'm* the mean one! Just tell him what happened!"

Jerry looked down.

"I sat on a tube of shaving cream," he mumbled.

I looked at Tricia. She shrugged.

"Okay, so you sat on the tube of shaving cream and the cap came loose and is in your rectum, correct?"

"Right! It's in my damn butt!" he spat.

"Okay. Anything else I need to know?"

He shook his head. I read the ER notes.

Gerald Guthrie, twenty, single, smokes a pack a day, drinks two to six beers a day, takes no medicines, has no allergies, no surgeries in the past.

"Looks like you're in pretty good health, Gerald," I surmised.

He said nothing.

"Goes by Jerry," Tricia said.

"Do you want to tell me anything, Jerry?" I asked again.

He shook his head.

"Okay. So you live alone, here in Hotspur, three blocks from the hospital, you work at the Argyris Garage and Body Shop on Commercial, you were in the shower and sat on a can of shaving cream some time this afternoon. The cap went inside your rectum."

Jerry grunted.

"The problem is, that's a smooth plastic cap with nothing really to grip," I added.

Jerry looked away.

"Then you called Tricia for help, drove out to her, and she tried to fish it out, but couldn't, and told you to come down here to the ER. You went ahead and she followed. Right so far?"

He nodded, surprised. I turned to Tricia.

"What I want to know is, what did *you* do?" I asked.

Tricia crossed her arms and stepped back.

"How the hell did you know that?" she asked. "His Royal Highness Lord Simon told you stuff in the corridor?"

"No. I read your addresses from your ER registration. Jerry lives nearby, and he said he saw me at noon, so he was home till at least noon, it started raining heavily around two. There's a lot of mud on his truck. You live in the country. I guess he came to see you first, you told him to come to the ER and followed him. Less mud on your truck, but it's all on the front and headlamps so you followed him closely."

"Okay, so what?" Tricia asked uncomfortably.

"So did you do something to get it out?" I asked.

Tricia looked away. Jerry groaned.

"I tried," she admitted.

"You did? How?" I was incredulous.

"Had a long scissors. Borrowed it from the hospital when I was here."

"You tried to get it out with *scissors?*" I asked, astounded.

"Blunt tipped scissors. That's all I had!" Tricia countered.

"Obviously you didn't get it out, but did you end up cutting the rim?"

"Yeah. Couple three times."

I slumped.

"So instead of a smooth lower rim, now there's a jagged rim!"

"That's why he's bleeding," Tricia explained.

"This goes from bad to worse," Simon declared.

"We need to send you to Abilene or Dallas or somewhere they can put in a scope and grab it with a forceps and pull it out," I said.

"I already called Abilene. They said no, it wasn't an emergency, and they didn't have a gastroenterologist who would accept the patient anyway," Simon said.

"Did you try Dallas?"

"Same story at Central, Holy Cross and Memorial," Simon said.

"Doesn't help he has no insurance," Tricia added. "Guess you're it!"

I paused.

"Do you have any other medical problems?" I asked Jerry.

He shook his head.

"I'm going to do a general exam first," I said.

A quick general exam was unremarkable, except for a stud in his tongue and a ring in his belly button.

"Okay, now I'm going to do a rectal exam. Is it okay to have Tricia in the room?"

Jerry nodded.

"Please roll over on to your left side and pull your jeans and underwear down, and bring your knees up to your chest."

I slipped on a pair of vinyl gloves and opened a sachet of lidocaine jelly. I noticed a small tattoo below his waistline: *Duke*.

"You want to attend Duke University?" I asked.

Jerry stiffened but said nothing.

"I'm going to put my finger in your rectum, through the anus, the hole where the bowel movements come out, okay?"

Jerry grunted.

"I'm using some numbing jelly, so it won't hurt so much in a few minutes."

There was bright red blood seeping out. I wiped it with gauze and cautiously inserted my finger. Jerry winced.

"I'm sorry. Don't mean to hurt you."

I felt the cap immediately. It was horizontal, about two inches long and three-quarter inches in diameter. The rim was cut and distorted. I pushed it and made it lie vertically. I waited to make sure it didn't flip back into its original position. I withdrew slowly.

There was a squirt of blood and there were blood clots on my finger.

"Something's happening!" Jerry warned.

There was a sudden spurt of yellow water, blood and bowel movements. It roared over the towels and splashed to the floor, splattering everything nearby. I jumped back. The stench of feces hit immediately.

"Tricia gave me some magnesium liquid, to make me crap it out," Jerry groaned.

"I'm sorry for screwing it all up," Tricia said.

Simon and I cleaned up the mess and mopped the floor quickly.

"How are you going to get it out, Doctor?" Simon asked.

He tossed the towels in a yellow bag and tied it up, but the smell remained. Simon sprayed air freshener.

"I call this new smell *shitrus*," he grinned. "Go on. How are you going to get it out?"

"I don't know. I could grasp the lower rim with a blunt forceps and pull down, but the rim will hit the anus and rip it. He won't be able to pass it, the anus is spasming and too narrow for that," I said.

"Is his rectal tone *normal?*" Simon asked. "I mean, he got the bloody thing in!"

"There's spasm from the trauma, so it's all pretty tight," I answered.

I covered Jerry with a fresh towel and sat down on a stool next to him.

"Get me a vaginal speculum, like we use for deliveries. I can hold the anus open with that," I ordered. Simon hurried off.

I sat and thought, then turned to Tricia.

"I've got a plan," I told her, "and I have an odd request."

"You mean, a queer request?" she shot back.

"Ha ha," Jerry said, bitterly.

"Can you get me some super glue?" I asked.

"Super glue? You mean the kind they use for repairs and such?"

"Yes," I answered.

"You want super glue?" she asked again. "You're not kidding?"

"I'm serious," I said.

"I can get some. Grocery's closed but let me make some phone calls. How many of those little tubes do you need?"

"Three or four."

"I'll get them. Grab me a smoke, too."

She left and we heard her drive away. Simon returned and handed me a sealed speculum set.

"So what's the plan?" he asked.

"I'm going to put more lidocaine on the anus, numb it up, then put in the speculum to keep the anus open. I'm going to put on a glove, put a little super glue on one fingertip, go through the speculum, and stick it on the rim. Once it hardens, I'll pull my finger out."

"So the finger tip of the glove is attached to the cap's rim and the rest of the glove is hanging outside the anus," Simon surmised.

"Yes."

"I get it," Simon nodded.

"I'll repeat it until I can cover the whole rim. Then I'll put a whole lot of lubricating jelly on the anus and pull on the gloves to get it out," I explained.

"So you protect his rectum from the cut-up rim by sticking vinyl glove tips on the outside of the rim?"

"Exactly."

"Could you rotate it? Do you think it went in at an angle?" Simon asked.

Jerry squirmed.

"It must have gone in at an angle, wouldn't you say?" Simon mused.

"No, it would have gone straight up. The rectum is vertical. In fact, the word rectum comes from the Latin word *rectus* which means straight."

"Wouldn't call him straight," Simon mumbled.

"Shut up! Just get it out!" Jerry snapped.

"Waiting on Tricia," I answered.

Simon stepped back and pointed to my feet.

"So the cap went straight in, but now it's diagonal. Interesting. By the way, your shoes and trousers got some direct hits!" he grinned.

I lost my temper. Those were my good shoes.

"I don't care *how* it got in, let's just get the damned thing out!" I snarled.

"That's what the actress said to the bishop," Simon quipped. Jerry laughed. Simon looked at me and winked.

Tricia returned with the super glue.

"Whoa! Smells like crap in here!" she announced cheerfully.

I inspected the tubes and handed them to Simon.

"Let me get ready," I explained. "I want to have a straight shot at the cap. I don't want to get stuck to the side walls."

Simon nodded. He removed the towel and exposed Jerry. He checked for residuals and wiped the skin clean. I pulled on a protective gown and face mask and double gloved. I wiped my shoes and slipped on shoe covers.

"Give me the speculum."

I sat down on the stool and rolled up to Jerry. I squeezed an inch of lidocaine ointment onto my finger.

"Jerry, I'm going to insert my finger into your rectum. It's going to hurt in the beginning, but I'm putting in some numbing ointment. The pain should get better in a few minutes."

There was more spasm the second time. I pushed gently, advancing gradually and holding as the resistance ebbed.

"That's really painful!" Jerry complained.

"I'm sorry."

"Can you give me a shot?" Jerry pleaded.

I hesitated.

"I know that Simon has an IV in you. If you still hurt in a few minutes, I'll give you some morphine."

"It's hurting a lot now!" Jerry repeated.

"I understand," I said. "Give it a few minutes."

"I can't stand the pain!"

I removed the speculum from the packet.

"That looks like a bird's beak!" Tricia said.

"The tapered end goes in and then I can spread the two parts, just like a bird opening its beak," I explained.

I moved the external lever that opened and closed the two curved blades of the speculum.

"He's going to deliver your baby!" Tricia chortled.

"Ha ha," Jerry answered.

"Want me to take a picture," Tricia inquired, "for your Christmas card?"

"Shut up! Give me a pain shot!"

Tricia signaled and moved to face Jerry.

"I got hooked on oxycodone on account of back pain. Six months later I was shooting it up. I used up all my veins. Arms, legs, feet, hands. Even tried my neck! Then I got real sick. I was sure I was going to die," she said.

Jerry shrugged, but listened.

"This here doctor found I had gotten an infection in my blood stream and it had gone to my brain and my eyes and heart. There was pus pockets inside my eyes!"

"You're lying!" Jerry mumbled.

"Pus pockets inside my eyes! I swear!" Tricia repeated.

"I'm going to insert the speculum," I warned.

"I had pus pockets deep inside my eyes! Dr. Mather saw them, that's how he knew what was going on! I was in Dallas and all the medical students came by to see me on account of my pus pockets!" Tricia said.

I inserted the speculum. Jerry winced, but said nothing. I pulled open the blades and locked them in place.

"Them pus pockets in my heart was sending bits of pus into my eyes and my brain. And everywhere! I was so sick, there was truckloads of bugs and germs in my blood!"

"Liar!" Jerry declared.

"I swear it! Pus and blisters deep in my eye, all the medical students coming down to look at them!" Tricia went on, gaining strength. "Ask him! What'd you call them, Doc?"

I pulled on gloves and dabbed superglue on the tip of a finger.

"Roth spots," I said. " They're called Roth spots."

I inserted my finger through the speculum and felt for the rim.

Jerry spun around.

"Yow! You're hurting me!" he yelped.

I quickly pinned the cap down and held pressure.

Jerry heaved and another torrent of yellow liquid burst out.

"Hold on, doctor," Simon said, and covered everything with towels.

I slipped off the glove and put on another. Simon applied another drop of superglue on the tip of the index finger. I held the speculum in place with my left hand and inserted my right index finger again. This time I found the hollow part of the cap.

Jerry howled.

"What are you doing?" he wailed. "It's hurting a lot!"

"I'm applying pressure. Hold still!"

"I can't! I can't! Stop this! It's hurting too much!" Jerry tried to sit up.

"Don't get up now! Lie down!" Simon ordered, and held him down.

I withdrew my finger from the glove.

Tricia came to my side.

"Jerry, you've got two plastic gloves coming out your butt!" she announced.

Jerry was confused.

"What the heck?" he said.

I removed the speculum and applied more lidocaine to the anus.

"Now he's putting some numbing salve on your butt!" she went on.

Jerry grunted.

"Nice round butt!" Tricia complimented.

Jerry was silent.

I pulled on the two gloves. The rim hit the anus, and Jerry cried out.

"Morphine! Give him four milligrams IV!" I ordered.

Simon injected it. We waited two minutes.

I tugged again. Jerry whimpered.

I twisted the gloves and pulled harder. Jerry cried out again, just as loudly.

"Four more milligrams of morphine!" I ordered.

Simon complied.

"Jerry, push down! Push down!" I said.

"As if you're having the biggest crap of your life!" Tricia added, helpfully.

Jerry strained. I pulled, with increasing force.

The gloves ripped off and Jerry screamed. There was a burst of blood and Jerry lashed out at Simon. Simon crashed to the floor and scrambled up.

"Bloody hell!" Simon said, and pinned Jerry down again.

I cleaned the anus with gauze. Three quarters of the lower rim was protruding. I whooped and pulled on fresh gloves and Tricia squeezed out the last of the superglue onto the sides of my little finger. I inserted it into the cap and pushed against the rim.

Jerry struggled to break loose but Simon pushed down harder.

I waited another two minutes for the glue to harden. It seemed like an eternity.

"Go for it, Doc!" Tricia urged.

I slipped my fingers out of the glove and tugged.

The cap came out half an inch, then popped back in.

I tugged again and grabbed it, but it slipped again.

"We're going to lose it!" I cried.

Jerry yelled and pushed down with all his might. I tugged again, struggling to keep the cap angulated correctly.

There was a loud pop and the cap shot out and hit the floor. Jerry howled. The orange cap tumbled on the floor, streaked with blood and feces and purple vinyl fragments. It slammed against the wall and shuddered.

"Good night!" Tricia said, in awe and relief. "Good *night!* All that effort for that crazy thing?"

Jerry mumbled and quickly drifted into sleep.

Simon and I cleaned up. The rectal bleeding stopped after ten minutes and we were soon getting Jerry ready for discharge.

"He should eat lots of soft fiber for the next week or so,"

I told Tricia, "pears, peaches, apples, beans, lentils, legumes."

"I'll make sure he eats a big bowl of beans every day," Tricia promised.

"There may be some bleeding when he has a bowel movement, but it should stop in a couple of days."

Jerry woke up.

"Thanks, Doc," he mumbled sheepishly. "Sorry you got shit all over your shoes."

"I can clean them," I answered.

"Jerry's pretty groggy," Tricia said. "I'll take him home. He can't drive."

"I can drive," Jerry protested.

"No, Tricia drives or you stay here," I ordered. "I know you live close by."

"Yeah? How do you know?" Jerry questioned.

"It was on your ER record, remember? And you saw me come to your neighbor's house for lunch, and they live close to the hospital."

Jerry scowled. He wagged a finger at me.

"That's right, I saw you. You went to Roger and Gwen Parrish's house for lunch today!" he said.

"Yes, they invited me. My family was away for Thanksgiving."

"You had a bottle of wine," Jerry went on. "You had a big old bottle of wine!"

"Yes?"

"Roger's a minister with the Church of Christ, Doc!"

I turned red.

"They don't touch any alcohol, Doc! What were you thinking?" Tricia asked, aghast.

"I didn't realize!" I stammered. Tricia shook her head in disbelief.

"Not so smart, eh?" Jerry crowed. "You screwed up too,

today, didn't you?"

I smiled.

"We all make mistakes," I admitted.

"Yeah," Jerry nodded. "We all make mistakes."

He draped an arm over Tricia's shoulder and they trudged out.

CHAPTER 4

THE FRIDAY NIGHT STORM

Maya and the girls returned from Canada on Friday afternoon. Anjali was not feeling well that evening. After dinner, she climbed in on my side of the bed, flung her arm and leg over me, and buried her face in my ribs. Priya scrambled onto Maya. All four of us huddled together in the cold, and gazed out the big window.

There was a power outage and the neighborhood was dark and silent. The window glimmered the graphite glow of twilight. A storm had just blown through, and another was coming. We watched as the trees swayed and straightened separately, then bowed again together; the bushes and yucca and oaxilla trembled, then were flung from side to side, and finally flattened as the furies gathered. Towers of dust and leaves slashed in and out like scythes. A gale grabbed leaves and dust, paper and pebbles and scraps, rolled them into fistfuls and flung them at us. The chain-link fence shuddered and the window rattled; the red bucket swing snapped off and was hurled into a corner. The trash can flew into the air and slammed into the fence, the contents and lid disappeared. The wind swept around and sucked its material back and attacked again. It pounded the walls, hammered the roof and gutters, and tugged at the doors, wailing and whistling and screaming.

The light faded to an inky gloom, sparing only the outlines of the tallest oaks and mesquites. The treetops swung back and forth more and more, then bowed down for minutes on end before snapping back upright. The raging winds slowed down abruptly and the trees stopped bending and simply stood and shivered as the eye of the storm thundered into Hotspur.

Bursts of rain lashed the windows and walls again and again like volleys of birdshot and crashed against the ceiling. Bolts of lightning exploded and flashed precise white fissures across the sky. The faint light then vanished completely and the murkiness made the violence unnerving. Priya and Anjali winced and shrank back further. Anjali gripped me tightly and whimpered. She felt very warm. Priya relocated in between Maya and me as Anjali squirmed away from the window. Slowly, the howling died down and the rain softened to a steady rattle.

Maya watched silently from the other end of the bed, lying down with her head propped up. Before I could tell her about Anjali's fever, Priya started talking about their adventures in Canada.

"We went skiing, Dad!" she gushed. "So much fun! Anjali and I and Tonya went down the bunny slopes, and we went so fast and didn't fall down even once!"

"Did Mom ski as well?" I asked.

"Yes! It was so exciting! Then we had bear claws! Do you know what bear claws are, Dad?"

"No," I admitted.

"They're big donuts, shaped like claws, covered in sugar! *So* good!"

"That sounds delicious."

"And we went to the CN tower and ate Chinese food and went to a big park and saw a movie and had popcorn!"

Priya was beaming in the dark.

"Missed you," Anjali mumbled.

"I missed you too! I'm so glad you're home!" I said.

"Were you busy?" Priya asked.

"Yes, it was busy. But I expected it. Hey, Mom said Anjali wasn't feeling well yesterday, and I think she's very warm right now. Maybe she's running a fever."

I turned to scrutinize Anjali. She threw her arm across my waist and buried her face deeper.

"I okay," she declared.

"Their money is called loonie, which means crazy!" Priya continued. "And their flag has a maple leaf because they have a lot of maple trees and because they like maple syrup and Pooja Auntie gave us some but they wouldn't let us take it through the airport so we went and gave it back!"

Priya paused for breath.

"Dad, will you tell us a story? An Akbar and Birbal story?" she asked.

"Yes, story," Anjali agreed.

"We haven't heard one for a whole week!" Priya pointed out.

Anjali was very warm. I worried that she had a fever. I wondered if I could find the thermometer and medicine in the dark.

"All right. Which one?" I said.

"The one about when the Queen wanted to replace Birbal with her brother," Priya suggested.

"That, that," Anjali nodded.

I cleared my throat and looked outside. It was darker than ever, nothing was visible, and the rain and wind rose back to a crescendo. It raged against the house, ripped off shingles, snapped the branches and hurled them, and raged across the county. There was a final fusillade of hail and rain and suddenly there was silence again.

We exhaled and sank back.

"Now tell the story, Dad," Priya pleaded.

I smiled. Priya was persistent.

"A long time ago in India, there was a great king," I started.

"Called Emperor Akbar," Priya cried.

"And he had a very clever Prime Minister."

"Called Birbal!"

"Called Birbal, yes. Emperor Akbar was very fond of Birbal because Birbal was very wise. But one day his wife, the Queen, complained to him and said, why do you always favor Birbal? You should make my brother, Sajid, your Prime Minister. The Emperor looked out the window of his palace and saw a caravan in the distance. He turned to his wife and said, I see a caravan to the east, far away. Send your brother, Sajid, to find out about it. So the Queen ran and told her brother."

"Then what happened?" Priya asked.

"Then the Queen's brother, Sajid, got on his horse and rode all the way to the caravan and talked to them and came back as fast as he could and told the Emperor, my lord, they are rice merchants from Bengal. And the Emperor said, what kind of rice do they have? Is it fine or coarse? And Sajid, the Queen's brother said, oh, I'm so sorry, I didn't ask that, but I'll go back and find out."

Anjali clucked in disapproval.

"So he got back on his horse and rode as fast as he could to the caravan and got the answer and came back," Priya continued, her voice slowing.

"Yes. He came back and said, Excellency, they have fine quality rice. And the Emperor said, how much do they have and how much do they want for it?"

"And the Queen's brother didn't know, so he got back on his horse and rode as fast as he could and asked the questions and came back again," Priya said, drowsily.

"Exactly. Then the brother returned and said, they have forty bushels of top quality rice and they want two silver mohurs per bushel. So Emperor Akbar asked, how much does rice usually cost? And the brother said, I'm sorry, I don't know."

I paused to check on the girls. Anjali was asleep, and still felt very warm. Priya was struggling to stay awake.

"Go on, go on," she insisted. "I'm not sleepy!"

I smiled. I had to hurry up.

"So Emperor Akbar asked Sajid to sit down and summoned Birbal. He told him, find out about that caravan there. Birbal was back in an hour."

Priya was silent.

"He said, your Highness, they are rice merchants from Bengal. They are selling basmati rice but I checked with a sieve and found they had mixed the long grain rice with short grain brown rice. There was no question of paying two silver mohurs per bushel, in fact I told them they should be punished. The current cost is one mohur per bushel for long-grain rice. We need rice for our army's campaign next week. So I bought their rice for half a mohur per bushel and they are delivering it to the granary right now."

Priya and Anjali were fast asleep. Maya spoke up.

"So Akbar smiled at his Queen and she said, I understand why you favor Birbal so much. He always thinks ahead and does not have to be told to do things," Maya finished, "unlike someone I know."

Anjali's crying woke me up. Maya and I jumped out of bed and raced to the bathroom. Anjali had vomited near the sink and was retching and crying. We wiped her face and mouth and changed her pajamas, and she vomited again. She didn't want to leave the bathroom. Maya squatted and steadied her. I wiped her down with warm water and brought her cold water to rinse; she refused. She tried sucking on frozen lemonade but retched again. She heaved and brought out some saliva and cried again.

She had a fever, so we lit two candles and gave her a tepid bath. She settled back in bed but looked ill and tired. She refused to drink anything.

Priya bustled back and forth, worried.

"She told me she didn't feel well this afternoon," Maya said.

"I think she's getting dehydrated," I said.

"What's that?" Priya asked.

"It means she needs fluids like water."

"Can't she drink water?"

"Not right now. Maybe later. But I don't want to wait."

"So are you going to give her a shot?"

"No, I think I should start an IV in her vein and give her some fluids. I see a good vein in her hand and I don't want to wait. If Anjali throws up more, she will lose more fluids and her veins will become thinner."

"Then you won't be able to start the IV?" Priya asked.

"Right."

Maya looked carefully at Anjali.

"She doesn't look that bad," Maya said, "but you're the doctor. If you feel she needs an IV, can you start it at home?"

"I'm sure I can get the IV material from the hospital," I said.

"Even with all the trouble?" Maya asked. "You know, with Dr. Ehrlich?"

"This is a personal thing," I said. "Even Dr. Ehrlich wouldn't stop me starting an IV on my own child. I'm going to go down to the hospital and pick up the supplies. I'll be right back."

I changed and turned the porch lights on in case the power came back. I stepped out and surveyed the damage. There were leaves and branches everywhere, and wide swathes were covered with sheets of mud, paper, shingles and wood siding. I locked the door and cleared the driveway of larger branches and sodden cardboard.

I drove down the hill slowly, avoiding the debris and a dog that lunged and chased me a block. The streets suddenly lit up as I approached the hospital; power was restored. I parked next to a white Lexus with gold lettering. My heart fell. Inside the car was a copy of the *Dallas Daily Chronicle*. The smell of diesel from the hospital's generator hung heavily.

I walked into the ER. Dr. Ehrlich was there, stitching up a facial laceration. Simon was assisting.

"What do you want?" Dr. Ehrlich snapped.

"My daughter's sick. I want to start an IV for her," I answered, in the same tone.

"Then bring her here, we will start one for her," Dr Ehrlich said, smoothly.

"No, I want to keep her home," I retorted.

"You're not on staff here anymore, perhaps you forgot?" he continued, looking down at the laceration and suturing it with elaborate slowness.

"I just want the supplies. I will take care of her at home," I said.

"Denied," Dr. Ehrlich said coolly. "Bring her here. No special treatment for you!"

Simon straightened up.

"Hold on! That's not fair!," he said.

"Not cricket, eh?" Dr. Ehrlich mocked.

"No," Simon said, "not by a long shot. Unfair!"

Dr. Ehrlich glared at him.

"Keep your mouth shut!" he snarled.

"Dr. Ehrlich, with all due respect, you're not being fair," Simon continued.

"I don't give a rat's ass!" Dr. Ehrlich snapped.

Simon stiffened and flushed.

"Keep pressure on the wound, you moron! Then give him a tetanus booster. I'm going to write some antibiotics for him," he ordered.

Dr. Ehrlich glared at me and retreated to the office and started dictating.

I was furious. I was determined to have my way. I walked away quickly to the nurses' station and sought out the charge nurse.

"Teresa, my daughter is ill. I think she has gastroenteritis and she's throwing up and can't keep anything down. She's getting dehydrated. I want to start an IV for her at home. Can you give me an IV start kit and a couple bags of dextrose saline?"

"Oh, bless her heart, poor thing! " Teresa said. "Of course, doctor!"

We gathered the material quickly.

"What sort of butterfly? Twenty-two gauge?" she asked.

Before I could reply, there was a commotion. Dr. Ehrlich rushed up to the nurses' station, his face purple.

"Stop! Stop right now!" Dr. Ehrlich grabbed Teresa's wrist roughly.

"Dr. Ehrlich!" Teresa protested, "you're hurting me!"

She dropped the butterfly needle. He turned and faced me, his face contorted.

"I already told him no! He deliberately disobeyed my orders! Deliberately!" Dr. Ehrlich roared.

Other nurses gathered and stood uncomfortably.

"Should I call Mr. Dawkins?" Teresa asked.

"Yes!" I said.

"No!" Dr. Ehrlich screamed, "that's an order! I'm in charge! David Dawkins is in Oklahoma!"

My heart sank. I remembered David telling me he was going to see his daughter.

I put the supplies down.

"Good!" Dr. Ehrlich declared.

There was nothing to say. The nurses looked bewildered. I thought of punching Dr. Ehrlich. I edged closer. He stepped back and held up his hand.

"Now go home!" Dr. Ehrlich said. "Bring her here!"

I stared at Dr. Ehrlich with utter hatred and bitterly regretted having saved him from the Gutierrez family. I wondered if I could take my words back and offer to assist in his prosecution. Before I could say anything, Simon appeared behind Dr. Ehrlich.

"Dr. Ehrlich, your patient Colton Waverly is ready to go home. I've given him a tetanus booster. May I discharge him?" Simon asked.

Dr. Ehrlich did not turn around.

"Yes, discharge him," he said, glaring at me. "I'm going to watch and make sure that Dr. Mathur leaves empty-handed."

"I'm going to see the patient to his vehicle, be right back," Simon went on cheerfully.

"Fine!" Dr. Ehrlich snapped.

Simon paused behind Dr. Ehrlich and held up a bulging white plastic bag that said *Patient Belongings* and winked at me.

"There's another patient in the ER. Six-year old with ear pain," Simon announced, "whenever you're ready, sir."

"I'm just saying goodbye to Dr. Mathur. I will return after he leaves the building."

Dr. Ehrlich crossed his arms and waited for me. He watched me as I withdrew. I dragged my feet, to allow Simon a head start. I stared longingly at the supplies at the nurses' station.

Dr. Ehrlich snatched them up and gleefully returned them to their shelves. I hung my head and headed out. As I left I heard Dr. Ehrlich berating the staff.

"In England, they do what they want, but this is different!" he bellowed. "We have rules! You can't just walk in and take hospital supplies, even if you're a doctor! This is not England or India!"

It was still raining lightly. I made my way to my red Corolla. The white plastic *Patient Belongings* bag was on my car trunk, discreetly out of view from the ER. It contained two bags of dextrose saline, three twenty-two gauge butterfly needles, two IV start kits, a tourniquet, tongue blades, alcohol wipes, tape, and a piece of paper that said *Commonwealth!*

I looked around the parking lot for Simon. He wasn't there.

Thank you, Birbal, I thought.

Anjali watched with fascination as I tied the tourniquet on her forearm and obligingly clenched her little fist. I cleaned the back of her hand with alcohol and a thin blue vein appeared. I held my breath and slid the needle in and she didn't flinch. I saw a crimson flash in the plastic tubing and exhaled. I quickly connected the IV tubing to the needle and the bag, and hooked the bag of dextrose saline on a hanger and hung it from the top of the bedpost. I splinted her wrist with the tongue blades so she wouldn't displace the needle if she moved her wrist. Priya watched with a hand over her mouth and blinked back tears.

I turned the lights out and watched the three of them fall asleep. Priya slept next to Anjali, her arm stretched over her sister. I remembered the day Anjali was born; Priya had been overjoyed and had often slept with her arm draped the same way. Anjali watched Priya's every move and imitated her all the time. She called Priya *didi*, which is Hindi for older sister. It was a close and happy relationship.

I sat on the floor with my back resting against the window and gazed at them. It was silent except for the drumming of rain. Half an hour later, it stopped raining and I listened to their breathing. I studied their lips and their noses and their fingers. The clouds cleared and moonlight crept in and gilded their faces; they lay like pharaohs. Their breathing grew slower and softer. I watched their chins lift and drop. Their breathing became a murmur, punctuated by the dripping of the gutters and the moaning of loosened metal. It was so peaceful.

I checked the IV to make sure it was dripping. I let the first bag go in over two hours and then set the second bag at a slower rate. I remembered the night Anjali was born, how I was fascinated by her and studied every feature of her face and hands and feet for hours, this creation of olive skin and sinew, with eyebrows and eyelashes and forehead and wisps of black hair.

Weariness returned rapidly. I stretched out and fell asleep on the floor, my back to the window.

Anjali slept well. She was up eating cheese toast and watching Sesame Street when I woke up. The IV was still dripping slowly, the plastic bag balanced on top of the recliner. I was aching and groggy. I inspected her hand. No swelling. I removed the splint, cleaned her hand with alcohol, and cautiously pulled the needle out. She tugged impatiently as I held her back and stuck a small bandage over the puncture site. She rushed back to her sister as if nothing had ever happened.

CHAPTER 5

LOVE THY NEIGHBOR

Priya peeled back Anjali's bandage and examined the needlestick site with awe as Anjali lounged and watched Sesame Street. I sat at the table and munched cheese toast and sipped coffee. Maya stuck her head out of the kitchen.

"Doris Marsh called this morning, around seven," she announced.

"Mrs. Marsh? You mean, our neighbor from across the street?"

"Yes, exactly. Guess why she called."

"She needed some help after the storm last night?"

"No, she called because she found out that Anjali was sick and wanted to bring over some home-made chicken soup," Maya said, smiling at my surprise.

"But she's very ill! She has severe heart disease and can barely walk!" I said.

"Listen to this. She called me first, then she actually came over in her golf cart! You were asleep. She zipped down, handed over two bottles of soup and shot back across the street to her garage, like a yo-yo," Maya explained.

I shook my head in disbelief.

"How did she know Anjali wasn't well?" I asked.

"I don't know," Maya answered, "but I said you would come by to return the soup containers this morning. I've washed and dried them."

I shrugged.

"Why not? I've got nothing else to do. I can't go to the hospital or clinic," I said.

"Don't be bitter," Maya said.

I showered and dressed quickly. The girls were still watching TV as I stepped out with the containers. The front yards and streets were littered and caked with drying mud, and the humid air hung heavily. I retrieved my stethoscope from my car and trudged across the street.

Mrs. Marsh answered the door. She was a thin, frail woman with bifocals and a halo of cropped white hair. She greeted me, turned her walker slowly, and shuffled behind it. She spoke as she retreated.

"You didn't have to return them so quickly!" she protested. "I'm in no hurry, you know!"

"I know," I answered, "but I was free and wanted to see you. I wasn't doing anything this morning."

"You were free? Oh, because that awful man from Dallas had you suspended?" she asked.

"Yes," I admitted.

"How does this affect you?"

"Well, I can't practice in the hospital until I'm cleared."

"How long will that take?"

"I don't know. Maybe a week or two."

"So you can relax with your family!" she smiled.

"Yes, but my contract with the hospital says I can't take leave for more than a week at any time. It clearly says I must provide medical services for the community continuously. But everything's in the hospital – the ER, the clinic, the in-patient ward."

"So they won't pay you?"

"I don't care about the pay. My application for a green card will be in jeopardy."

"I see," Mrs. Marsh said, and sat down in a large armchair. She waved to another.

The living room was long and rectangular. The long wall facing the garden was mostly sliding glass panels, and looked out over a border of trim Bermuda grass and two cast-iron bird feeders, after which the hill fell away, revealing an aerial view of the village of Hotspur, a lattice of brown and white brick and plywood houses, mottled black roofs, silver carports and blue trampolines. Muscular trucks navigated the crossword of roads and clothes and carpets dried out between clusters of oaks, pecans and mesquites. Mrs. Marsh's back yard was active: red cylinders with perches hung from tree branches, and hummingbirds swooped around them. They sucked sugary water and darted off. Blue jays and magpies waddled and nodded as they inspected the wet turf, and jabbed and swooped after escaping insects.

"I love the view," she said. "I spend *hours* looking outside."

"I like your hummingbird feeders."

"They're made here in Hotspur. The owner found out that hummingbirds prefer small red flowers and he measured their beaks and created the ideal feeding base with red flowers and perfect holes in their centers."

I nodded.

"I was looking for the hospital."

"It's over there to the left, hidden behind the trees on Pecan and behind the Land Bank and Argyris Garage."

"Yes, I see it now. You do have a great view."

"Do sit down! Would you like a cup of tea?" she asked.

I smiled.

"I could tell from your accent that you were from England," I said.

"Yes, I'm English. Married my Bennie when I was twenty-one. He was a Yank, you know, come over for the war."

"There were a lot of Americans in England, weren't there, towards the end of the war?"

"Yes. We didn't like them at first, you know. They were overbearing, overfed, and over here, people said," she laughed.

"But you obviously found one you liked."

"True."

"Do you ever think of going back to England?"

"Well, I used to. Of course, I can't now, but before that I didn't want to because my three boys were here and Bennie was so busy on the ranch."

The kitchen was separated from the living room by a half-wall. I went to one of the cupboards.

"I've been here before so I know where the tea bags are. You still use PG tips?" I asked.

"Of course! Unless I can get some Ty-phoo!" she said.

"You only get an *ooh* with Ty-phoo," I said, remembering the jingle.

Mrs. Marsh laughed and nodded.

I poured boiling water into the cups and added the tea bags.

"You seem to be walking comfortably," I noted.

"I am," Mrs. Marsh replied. "I followed your advice and reduced my water. I thought I was supposed to drink eight glasses of water a day!"

"No, that's not for everyone. You can get too much of a good thing. Even water."

"Even water? I always thought you could never get enough water," she said.

"Even water. Have you ever over-watered a plant?"

"Yes."

"So you know that too much water *can* be bad."

"So how much water is right?"

"Whatever makes you pass urine every four or five hours in the day, and doesn't make your blood tests get messed up," I answered. I lifted the sugar pot so she could see it.

"One spoon, please. That's lovely," Mrs. Marsh said.

I added milk and sugar.

"I've got a tin of shortbread biscuits there," she added.

I placed everything on a tray and set it on a nearby ottoman. We sipped tea and surveyed the town below.

Mrs. Marsh dipped her shortbread in her tea and nibbled.

"How did you know Anjali was ill?" I asked.

"My nephew, Simon, works in the Emergency Room," she explained.

I nodded.

"I knew he was from England," I said, "but I didn't know about this connection."

"He came over to visit me for a holiday and fell in love. With a foreign country and with a sweet young lady."

"Just like Bennie did."

Mrs. Marsh nodded and smiled.

"He's a *very* nice boy, my Simon," she declared.

"Simon helped me a lot last night," I said. "He let me have the supplies I needed to start an IV for Anjali. That way I didn't have to take her to the ER at night."

"Simon told me about it. He said you were upset."

"I was angry with Dr. Ehrlich. He was the one who started this mess. He blamed me for it and suspended me pending an inquiry. But I have a real problem waiting for this inquiry. If I can't see patients in the hospital then I'm in violation of my contract. Everything's in the hospital – the ER, the in-patients, the clinic!"

"So you need to get back in the hospital."

"Correct."

"Let me call some friends," Mrs. Marsh said. "Let's try to get this business over. I'm sure you did nothing wrong."

"The delay is not here in Hotspur but in Austin. We need

an independent expert to come down. They haven't set that up yet."

"Oh, fiddlesticks! I don't know anyone in Austin!"

I smiled.

"Actually, I came over to return the soup containers and to check on you. I see that your ankles are a lot less swollen. That's good. If you would lie back in your recliner, I could check your neck veins to see if they're still engorged."

Mrs. Marsh fussed and finished her tea. She pulled the lever and inclined back until she was at forty-five degrees.

"Your jugular veins are not as distended! That's good. Now let me listen to your heart and lungs."

She sat up straight.

"Breathe normally."

I listened carefully. There was a soft blowing murmur over her aortic valve, just to the left of the sternum.

"Now lean forwards, take a big breath and blow it all out."

She complied.

"Now hold your breath!"

I heard a new murmur, right after the aortic valve closed, like a short gasp.

"Breathe normally for a minute. Then let's do that again."

Mrs. Marsh breathed rapidly for a few minutes to catch up.

"Big breath in, breathe all the way out, then hold, hold, *hold* your breath!" I ordered.

I heard it again. There was a new murmur, just after the valve closed. Then I listened to her lungs. They were clear.

"What is it?" Mrs. Marsh asked.

"I'm not sure," I began.

"Tell me!" she insisted.

"Could be nothing."

She grasped my wrist.

"Tell me!"

"I hear a new murmur."

"What does that mean?"

"I'm not sure. I'm not a cardiologist."

"But what do you *think* it means?"

"The aortic valve, the valve that wasn't opening properly, is now not closing properly either."

"That's because of the calcium building up?"

"Yes. The valve becomes more rigid and brittle and leaks."

Mrs. Marsh looked away.

"Not a good sign, then," she surmised.

I was silent. She looked at me.

"Oh, come on! You can say it!" she smiled.

"I'm not a cardiologist," I repeated.

"My cardiologists in Houston said this would happen. And so it has. But they predicted I would be dead in six months, and that was two years ago. Aortic stenosis is what I have. What's this new murmur called?"

"Aortic regurgitation."

She dipped her shortbread thoughtfully.

"Aortic regurgitation," she repeated. She waited too long and the shortbread dissolved.

"You've done remarkably well, though!" I said.

She drained her tea and sat the cup down. She looked out silently for a few minutes.

"Do you ever think of death, doctor?" she asked.

"Sometimes," I admitted.

She looked out at the bird baths and the trees.

"I love looking at the trees and those bird baths," she said, "and I find it so strange to think that they'll still be here, exactly the same, even after I'm gone. And the wind chimes will be there and the hummingbird feeders and the house and the town and the sky and everything. Dear, dear Hotspur will still be here, after I'm gone. The day of my funeral, the week after my funeral, a year after my funeral. As if nothing really happened."

"It's sobering."

"I've grown accustomed to the fact that any day may be my last one," she said. "Sometimes I look up at the sky and ask, *when, God, when?* And when I get an answer, I say, *what, already?*"

I laughed.

Mrs. Marsh chuckled, "I still get shocked when I hear bad news. I know I shouldn't. Every day is a gift. Maybe that's why it's called the present."

I nodded.

"Every day is a gift, I should know," she went on. "May I tell you a story?"

I turned to face her.

"Go ahead."

"You're not in a hurry?"

"I've been fired," I shrugged. "I'm free."

She nodded.

"I remember the day I went to meet my Bennie at the train station to introduce him to my family," she said. "It was during the War. We had met near London, at Bletchley Park. He was an American liaison officer. We had grown very fond of each other and he was coming to meet my parents and sister, Agnes."

"In London?"

"No, we lived in a town called Coventry. It was in 1940. I was twenty years old. I wanted to marry him."

She blushed.

"That was *ages* ago. I went to the railway station in Coventry to receive him. It was the fourteenth of November, fifty-six years ago. He was twenty-two."

"What happened?"

"First, they said his train was delayed. While I waited, some German planes came over and dropped some ordnance and left. Well, I said to myself, thank goodness that's over. They probably meant to bomb London."

"That's why the train from London was delayed?"

"No. Those planes were just preparing for the bombers that followed. They started bombing Coventry that day and we couldn't stop them. First, they bombed the water pumps and the telephone system and the roads and the power supply so that we couldn't get help and the fire brigade couldn't put out any fires. Then they dropped bombs that blew the roofs off the factories and houses and finally they dropped incendiary bombs that went straight inside and burned everything down to the ground. Even the cathedral! *The cathedral!* And the bombers flew back and reloaded and hit us again and again, all night long. It was the worst night of my life, doctor. The air was thick and grey and full of burnt flesh and gunpowder and smoke and the screams went on and on, horrible screams and children wailing and sirens and the earth shook and buildings crashed. The screaming only stopped when there was another explosion. I tried not to cry but I couldn't hold back and I howled and howled and collapsed. I ran into the fires, I couldn't see anything. I was sure I would die."

I listened silently.

"What happened to your family?"

"We lived in Council housing. Our street was devastated. No one survived. Mother died that night, Father a week later. We never found Agnes."

"What happened to her?"

"I think she went to help and died in a fire, there were so many incendiary bombs, so many bodies were burnt beyond recognition. Even infants and children! They looked like little charred logs, doctor! Coventry reeked of sulfur and tar and skin and hair for weeks."

"Did Bennie get there later?"

"No, he had been held up in Bletchley Park. I think they knew something big was going to happen in Coventry and delayed him on some pretext."

"Why didn't they tell everyone if they knew about the raid?"

"They didn't want the Germans to know they had cracked the code, the Enigma code, you know, the code the Germans used for all their communications."

"So they sacrificed Coventry? To keep a secret?"

She nodded.

"I think so. I don't think that's the official version, but *I* think so."

"So did Bennie ever come to Coventry?"

"No, it was too painful. I went back to Bletchley Park after Father died and never returned. We married in London. Do you see those bird baths?"

"Yes."

"Bennie was bringing them as a gift for my parents; they loved birds. So we brought them here and I see the blue jays and mockingbirds and chickadees and pigeons and squirrels enjoy them every day."

I gazed at the bird baths with renewed interest. They were ribbed grey metal, streaked with ribbons of rust and speckled with mildew.

"Bennie found them in Camden. I love them. We had a beautiful bird bath in a park near our house, and Agnes and I used to feed the birds there when we were little."

A magpie dropped into one and wet its feathers and splashed. It stood up, flapped its feathers, and turned around.

"A thing is just a *thing* until you understand it's significance, yes? And every day is a gift," she repeated. "That's why it's called the present."

"So you have lived all these years, beating the odds in Coventry, marrying and moving to America, having children, and beating the odds in Houston?" I asked.

"Yes. I survived the fires and bombing of Coventry and expect to die in a sweet, calm part of Texas, looking out over my garden, at birds playing in my bird bath, in my home, and not in a hospital. Doctor, I'm ready whenever the good Lord wants me."

"There's a line somewhere in Shakespeare, Julius Caesar, I think, where Caesar says, *death, a necessary end, will come when it will come*," I said.

She nodded.

"Cowards die many times before their deaths; the valiant never taste of death but once," she quoted.

She clapped and turned sharply towards me.

"I called one of my doctors in Houston to give him an update, well, really to shock him and tell him I wasn't dead, and do you know what his staff said?" she asked.

"What?"

"He died a month ago. Pancreatic cancer. Woke up one fine morning with jaundice. Died three months later." She shook her head, "Life's just unpredictable, Doctor."

I looked at her keenly. She looked back and smiled.

"I know I don't have too much time left. This new murmur is another warning. But you know what, Doctor? I've had a good life. I'm grateful."

I nodded. She exuded calmness.

"I've been very fortunate. I haven't been in any pain. Just short of breath when I exert too much," she said.

"I understand."

"I've been fortunate. In Coventry, I was at the railway station when they bombed my home, and I survived. In Houston,

I was about to go for heart surgery, actually, when I went to buy my surgeon a gift card, and bumped into my internist. He was from India, too, by the way. He told me that his mother had atrial fibrillation, and was advised surgery to correct it. They were going to fix a valve that was failing, I forget which valve, but nevertheless, she had the surgery and then had complication after complication. She spent the next two years in hospitals and rehabilitation. She died in her sleep two days before she was to finally go home. She had been a very strong and active lady, and my internist says she would have probably done just fine without the surgery."

"So you changed your mind?" I asked.

"Yes. I think that things happen for a reason. I think my internist was there in that shop at that time for a reason," she answered.

She raised her head and spoke up in a different tone.

"I *do* hope Anjali is feeling well. I was *so* concerned about her!" she declared.

I returned the tea tray to the kitchen.

"She looked fine this morning. Amazing how quickly children recover!" I said.

I walked back to Mrs. Marsh.

"I had better get back. Thanks a lot for the soup. I'll make sure Anjali gets it. Remember, soup has a lot of salt, so *you* should go easy on it. It can overload your heart and lungs."

Mrs. Marsh looked at me with concern.

"Bangers and bacon too?" she asked.

"You mean, sausages? Sorry, too much salt."

"Potato crisps?"

"No."

"If it tastes good, spit it out?"

"Just be sensible."

"Ye Gods, I hope there's no salt in chocolates!"

"Hershey's chocolates will be fine."

"Cadbury's chocolates. American chocolates have more wax, because America is warmer than Britain."

I saw an opportunity.

"May I quote you? America is *warmer* than Britain?"

Mrs. Marsh was delighted.

"I meant no such thing! Impertinence! Such impertinence!" she trilled. "These Colonies are so revolting!"

"I'll lock the door on my way out." I said, and headed out.

Mrs. Marsh waved.

"Now remember to bill me for this visit! Medicare pays for home visits!"

Her parting words hovered in my mind as I cleared her driveway. Suddenly, their importance struck me.

Home visits?

Home visits!

I suddenly realized I could provide medical services to the people of Hotspur by doing home visits! I didn't need to be on staff at the hospital! I could still save my contract!

CHAPTER 6

HORSE THIEVES GULCH

David Dawkins was delighted.

"Home visits! Good night, I never thought of that! Yeah, Doc, that'll work!" he agreed. "Just keep on doing home visits till everything's cleared up. I'm going to call the lawyer to check, but, heck, I don't see a problem!"

"My contract only says I have to provide medical services to the community without interruption, I just checked it," I said.

"You sure?"

"Of course I'm sure! I just read it twice!" I said.

David grinned.

"Not many people actually *read* the contract!" he observed.

"My family's future depends on the next few months."

"You don't want to go back to India?" David asked, teasing.

"I don't want to be pushed around. I don't mind going back to India or London or anywhere, but not because of some bully."

"And our little Mrs. Marsh has shown us the way!" David said.

"Yes."

David rubbed his hands happily.

"Yes, yes! Oh, this is good! Just keep seeing patients in their homes, they'll love it and you're back on track!"

I nodded.

"We need to keep checking with Austin. I need to get back on staff," I pleaded.

"On it. How *did* Mrs. Marsh think of it?" he wondered. "I'm kind of pissed that I didn't think of it myself."

"I went to check on her. I went over her history and

medicines and examined her. When I was leaving, she told me to bill Medicare because that was basically a home visit."

"She's right! Medicare does cover home visits! Most doctors are too busy to do them, but you, seeing as you've been fired, that's perfect! Got nothing else to do when you're *fired!*"

"Thanks."

I stomped through the wet parking lot to my car, wondering how I would get the word out about home visits. I heard a booming voice.

"Hey, you there!"

I stopped.

"You in the white coat! You the doctor?"

I turned.

There was a man twice my size. He was at least six and a half feet tall and weighed over two hundred and fifty pounds. He pulled off his hat and extended a hand the size of a brick.

"Bill Hennessy!" he boomed.

We shook violently.

"Pleased to meet you. I'm Dr. Mathur."

"My pleasure entirely. Doc, I need you to come see my friend, Herschel. He's real sick, can't breathe, coughing up blood and stuff, looks like death warmed up!"

"If he's that sick, he should come here to the ER, where we can do more for him," I said.

Bill shook his head.

"Nope, not happening. Herschel hates hospitals. I begged him. Said he'd rather die than come to town. Says black folks ain't welcome in this town, and he's wrong, but he's stubborn as a mule."

I was at a loss.

"So where is he?"

"Out on the ranch. Just past Horse Thieves Gulch, before

the Bloody Basin. I'll take you right now. You ready?" Bill waved towards his truck.

"How far away is it?"

"Not far. Twenty miles out," Bill said, shrugging.

"Let me leave a message for my wife, I'll be right back."

Bill nodded and walked to his truck. I noticed that he walked with a limp, leaning to the left.

I went back to the ER. Simon was there.

"Doctor Mathur! You're back!" he exclaimed. "How's little Anjali?"

"Much better, thank you," I said. "Thanks for the supplies."

Simon shrugged.

"Have you sorted out your hospital status?"

"No, not really. I'm still suspended from the hospital. The case is dragging on. I'm just here to call home and tell them I'm going with this Bill Hennessy guy who wants me to go to his ranch near Horse Thieves Gulch and see his friend."

"So you're going to do a home visit?"

"Exactly. The inspiration came from your aunt, Mrs. Marsh. I can do home visits and not breach my contract."

"Brilliant! Mr. Hennessy was just here, looking for you."

"He found me. Do you know him?"

"Everyone knows him. They have a pretty big ranch out there, next to the Rhone ranch, past the Templar land. He was here in the ER some time back. I wasn't on call that night, don't quite know the details."

"I need to use the phone."

"Go ahead. Dr. Ehrlich isn't here."

I called home repeatedly. No one picked up.

"My wife must have taken the girls to Dairy Queen for French fries," I said. "It's a family ritual after someone's been sick and has recovered."

"No problem. I'll call her in a few minutes and let her know."

"Thanks, Simon."

I returned to Bill. I wondered whether it was safe to go off with him to an unknown destination. I pictured the police notice, MISSING: *small Indian doctor last seen climbing into gigantic white truck.*

I pulled myself up into the cab. It had two steps.

"This is a massive truck!" I declared. "It has double wheels on the back!"

"It's called a dually. Never heard of it?"

"No."

"When you're hauling stuff, Doc, you got to have a real truck. This is a restored Ford round cab. Five lights on top. It's a beauty!"

The interior was beige leather. The steering wheel and gear stick were custom-wrapped in matching tones. I strapped my seat belt and settled in. It smelled of cigars and air freshener.

"My first truck, it was a hauler in the oil field. Real bad shape. Windows fell down when we hit a bump, electricals shorted all the time, couldn't change gears without getting a shock! Damn door swung open if I hung a right!" Bill recalled.

We laughed.

"Yeah, but it taught me a lot about truck repair. Then I restored this one. Original everything, even the leather and mats."

I looked at my foot mat. It was immaculate. I noticed that Bill's floor mat was missing.

We drove for ten minutes in silence. We got on the highway to Abilene and accelerated.

"I love this land," Bill said

"It's got a rough beauty," I agreed.

"I love this land," Bill repeated. "Means everything to me. My daddy raised my brother and me here."

"Your dad was a rancher?"

"Kind of. Wasn't the way he was raised. Was raised in Boston and was a real good baseball player. He was offered a contract by the Red Sox, he was that good!"

"So he played for the Red Sox?"

"Nope. he turned them down. Enlisted instead. When he got back from the war, they had all moved on. My mother inherited this land in Texas so we all moved down."

"And you've been here ever since?"

Bill nodded.

"Daddy worked here till the day he died. Fell off some rocks, hit his head, bled around his brain. Helicopter couldn't get here fast enough. Least, he died on his own land doing what he wanted."

I nodded.

"See those ant hills?" Bill pointed out.

"Yes."

"Daddy always told me, those are the oldest farmers in the world, those ants. Grow some kind of a fungus in those hills, cathedrals they call them, grow some fungus and eat that fungus. They eat what they grow."

We swung off the highway and went up a dirt road. Bill stopped in front of a closed metal gate. He got out and I followed. Bill lifted a latch and unlocked it. The gate posts were twisted and the gate was buckled outwards, towards the highway.

"Watch out for the cattle guard!" he warned.

I looked down. There was a long ditch in front of the gate, and it was spanned by a small bridge made of metal tubes. The tubes were parallel to the gate, with spaces between the tubes.

"So the spaces in between are to stop the cattle from getting out?" I asked.

"You got it!" Bill replied. "Now be real careful with that gate, Doc! Don't twist your ankle!"

We opened the gate carefully.

"See that big black burn mark there on the side?"

"Yes."

"Rattlesnake was hiding there, just underneath. Threw some gasoline on it and lit a match. Dang rattlers!"

Bill drove in and I closed the gate behind us.

We passed stretches of golden grass and clusters of thorny leafless mesquite trees, agave, and cacti. There were several ponds, some with little water left.

Bill shifted and adjusted his foot. The truck jerked.

"Let me make a guess. You broke your ankle recently? The right one?" I said.

Bill flashed me a smile.

"Yes, that's right. Still hurts. Guess you seen me limping."

"You must have broken it pretty badly. I think you were bleeding a lot!"

Bill slowed down and turned to look at me.

"That's true, I did. How'd you know that?"

"Simon said you were in the ER some time back. It must have been something serious, otherwise you would never come. It was your right ankle so you had a hard time driving your truck. I guess it happened here on your ranch and you managed to get yourself into your truck. But you couldn't get out of your truck to open your gate so you rammed it."

Bill laughed.

"The gate come a whopper! How did you know about the gate?"

"Gate was buckled outwards. So you must have hit it

coming from inside."

"How'd you know about the bleeding?"

"Your floor mat is missing."

Bill chuckled.

"Yep, I bled something fierce all over it. Okay, Sherlock, tell me this: how come there's no damage to my front lights if I hit the gate?"

"You had a cattle guard on the front of the truck, I guess."

Bill laughed and punched my shoulder.

"Well, we have a real live Sherlock Holmes here, don't we now?"

It was a small two-bedroom wooden house with peeling green paint surrounded by mesquites and pecans. Part of the roof had caved in. Several windows were broken or boarded and the remaining ones were opaque. The pathway was covered with leaves and fallen pecans. Withered nettle grass and clusters of yaupon holly encircled the house like a garland. We walked up to the covered patio and let ourselves in.

"Hey, Herschel! Herschel!" Bill called.

The house was dark and cold and smelled like rotten meat. Bill shivered and turned on the lights. We entered a small living room with two wooden chairs and a coffee table covered with crumpled wet clothes. The floor was green shag carpet with bare patches near the doors. Bill pointed to the clothes on the coffee table.

"Laundry," he explained, "for me to do later."

The clothes reeked with the onion smell of hardened sweat and were streaked with dried sputum and blood.

"*Herschel!*" Bill repeated.

There was no answer. We walked into one of the two rooms on the right.

There was a tall, thin African-American man sitting up in

bed, with a bath towel in his hands, breathing rapidly. He wore shorts and nothing else. His chest glistened with sweat and the skin between his ribs sucked in with every breath. His shoulders rose and fell quickly and he pursed his lips tightly, whistling softly as he exhaled, holding each gulp of air as long as he could to scavenge every last molecule of oxygen. He held up a hand wearily. He paused a second then coughed hard into the towel, a wet and bubbly cough, heaving and contorting. He straightened and spat out the last dregs. He examined the towel with disgust. There was a putrid yellow smear with drops of blood.

Bill exhaled and stared.

"Thought you might be dead," he said cheerfully.

"Too mean!" Herschel shook his head. "Too mean - to die."

He leaned over the edge of the bed and hacked again.

"Got to – corruption – out!" he gasped.

Bill turned on the light.

"You look like crap," he said pleasantly.

Herschel ignored him.

"I got the doctor!" Bill added.

Herschel shook his head.

"No money!" he whispered.

"Don't worry about that! You need to be in the hospital!" I said.

I took out my stethoscope and approached. He waved me away.

"No place – for blacks!" he gasped.

I turned on the table lamp and looked at him. He was a gaunt, middle-aged man, with a sheen of fuzzy white hair all over his head. He was sweating and shivering, and breathing rapidly. His pulse was a hundred and twenty and he was hot.

"You've got a fever, and you look septic!" I said.

Herschel leaned forwards and wheezed.

I listened to his lungs from the front and back. There was good air movement on the left side but there were loud crackles on the right side.

"Sounds like peeling Velcro, every time you breathe! Can you say *one-one-one*?"

He looked at me, confused.

"Just say *one-one-one*," I repeated. "I want to see how sound travels through your lung."

He looked at Bill. Bill shrugged. Herschel gazed at me, his red eyes swollen and defiant.

"Let me explain. If you've got pneumonia then your lung tissue will be solid rather than like a soft sponge. When you say one-one-one, your words will sound louder. Solids conduct sound well. If you've got a fluid collection, they will sound softer, because fluids around the lung muffle the sound," I explained.

"Doc thinks he's some kind of detective," Bill said.

Herschel waited a few seconds and said, "One-one-one!"

I heard the sound boom through his right lung, magnified.

"Sounds like consolidation! This is pneumonia!" I declared.

I tapped in between his ribs on the back. It was soft on the left side, but hard as a stone in the lower three spaces on the right.

"You've got a big pneumonia on the right and there's some fluid there as well! You really need to come to the hospital!"

Herschel looked away and shook his head.

I looked at Bill. Bill threw his hands up in despair.

I felt something brush against my ankle. I stepped back hastily.

"Do you have a cat?" I asked.

Herschel shook his head.

"You used to have a cat," Bill said. "Maybe it's come back."

Herschel shook his head.

"I felt something move past my ankle. There's something underneath the bed. Maybe the cat came back. Bill, let's get Herschel to the main room. I want him to lie face down on the coffee table and I'm going to thump his chest to get the sputum out. Can we get some steam?"

Bill burst into action. He pulled Herschel off the bed and they staggered into the main room. I threw the clothes on a chair and laid a pillow on the table. Bill helped Herschel lie down on it, his chest resting on the pillow, and his face dangling down over the end of the table. Herschel grasped the sides of the table for support and started coughing immediately. I went to the kitchen on the other side of the living room and found a kettle. I filled it and set it to boil.

"Doc, you deal with that water, I'm going to see what's under the bed," Bill called out. "Maybe Herschel's cat came back."

He disappeared. I poured boiling water into two large pans and set them in the living room near Herschel's head. I recalled the anatomy of the right lung, with its three lobes, and how they drained. I pummeled the right side, starting at the base and working my way up. Herschel convulsed.

"Stop!" he protested, his face congested and red. He tried to get up but was too weak.

"Let me try! I'm trying to get the infection out!" I insisted and thumped the back of the chest again.

"Hurts!" Herschel protested.

I stopped for a minute, worried I had broken a rib.

"You were an athlete, weren't you?" I remembered.

Herschel gurgled and paused.

I seized the opportunity. I thumped again with greater vigor.

Herschel suddenly arched his back off the table. His body was racked with spasms and he drew up his arms and legs.

I held him on the table and prevented him from rolling off.
"Bill! *Bill*," I yelled, "I need you here!"

There was no answer.

Herschel arched up again and I pinned him down. He retched and gasped and grabbed at his throat. He twisted his face up towards me. It was swollen, dripping with sweat and his eyes bulged in pain.

He collapsed in a heap back on the table and produced a loud whistling sound. He thrashed from side to side. He lurched off the pillow, threw me off balance, and crashed to the floor. I fell back and hit the chair.

The room suddenly filled with the smell of vomit. Herschel threw up all over the carpet. The pillow fell into the pool of vomit. Herschel rolled towards it and hacked up a cupful of thick, amber, blood-stained pus directly onto his pillow. Bill swung open the door and stepped in from outside.

"Look at that crap!" Bill boomed with delight. "If that isn't the crappiest crap I ever saw! Like dog vomit!"

All of us gazed in awe at the congealed frothy mass that spread over the pillow and trickled down the edges.

"Hey man, good thing your carpet's already green," Bill declared.

Herschel took a few deep breaths and looked at me in surprise.

"You feel better?" I asked, trying to sound nonchalant.

"Uh-huh," he whispered.

Bill helped him stand and sat him in the other chair. We used the hot water to clean the vomit off the carpet. I opened the window and Herschel protested.

"I'm going to put him back in his bedroom," Bill said. "I saw what you did there. I'll come back and do it for him. I'm going to try to not bust his ribs!"

I watched Herschel. He looked a little better. He was breathing more comfortably. I knew he couldn't tolerate any more chest percussion.

"The lungs drain up towards the throat, like two bottles side by side," I explained, "and infection tends to settle at the bottom of the infected lobe. So sitting up and coughing just won't get the pus out from the bottom. You have to be lying flat, or even with your head low, to drain the pus."

"Makes sense, Doc," Bill said. "Maybe I can lift him up by his ankles and smack him like a baby!"

Herschel shook his head. He looked better.

"You - just try!" he rasped.

"Your breathing has improved. You're taking deeper breaths and not breathing as fast," I said.

"So you fixed him, Doc!" Bill enthused.

"Not yet. He needs medicines. I am going to write some antibiotics and some steroids for him and an inhaler. That should help. He needs to repeat the chest percussion thrice daily," I said.

"I'll take every chance I can get to beat the crap out of him," Bill said.

Herschel managed a weak grin.

The drive back seemed shorter. We opened and closed the gate together, and sped home.

Bill took off his hat and showed me a scaly rash extending along the edge of his hairline.

"Doc, when I went to the ER with my busted ankle they gave me antibiotics to prevent the bone from getting infected. But every time I get antibiotics, I get this darned rash, Doc! Look! All over my scalp!"

"Does it itch?"

"Itches like crazy!"

"So what have you taken for it?"

"They usually give me some high dollar creams and pills, Diflucan or something."

"It's a fungal rash. Normally, we have both bacteria and fungus on our skin, but antibiotics just wipe out the bacteria," I explained. "But antibiotics don't kill fungus. They only kill the bacteria that normally keeps the fungus in check."

"I'll be darned! So that antibiotic junk frees up fungus? That's why I get this rash, the fungus breaks loose?" Bill asked.

"That's it."

"Hate taking all those medicines. Last time it cost me four hundred dollars for that anti-fungus mess!"

"Do you want to try an old-time remedy?" I asked.

"Shoot, yeah!" Bill shot me a surprised look.

"Vinegar."

"Vinegar? You mean, like plain vinegar?"

"Yes."

"Kills fungus?"

"Kills a lot of fungus. You can try it on your scalp."

"Won't it burn?"

"Probably, but it works and it's a lot cheaper and simpler."

We reached the hospital parking lot and parked next to my Corolla.

Bill suddenly reached over and stuffed two hundred-dollar bills into my coat pocket.

"I don't want the money!" I protested.

Bill ignored me. He reached into his breast pocket and pulled out a roll of newspaper, and thrust it into my hands.

"What's this?"

"A memento of your visit," Bill grinned.

I began to unwrap it.

"It's what was under the bed," he said.

I looked up, startled.

"What was under the bed?" I asked.

Bill grinned.

"A rattlesnake. Don't worry, it was cold, they're not real dangerous when they're cold. Just grabbed it and took it out and killed it."

"So that's the rattle in here?" I asked, apprehensively.

Bill chuckled.

"Yes sir-ee. *Now* you *really* got a tail to talk about, Doc!"

CHAPTER 7

RODEO DRIVE

It was a cheerful Sunday afternoon. Maya and the two girls and I were driving on the highway north of Hotspur towards Abilene. Priya spoke up, although she already knew the answer to her question.

"Where are we going?" she asked, pleasantly.

"We're going to see a very nice lady called Mrs. Rutherford," Maya said. "She called us last Sunday and invited us to the Cattlewomen's Ball. Everyone's supposed to wear boots and jackets, and I told her I didn't have any. So she said I could borrow hers."

"Why do you want her jacket and boots?" Priya asked. "Why don't you just buy your own?"

"There's not enough time. The Ball is next week."

"Is it too expensive and Daddy doesn't have money?" Priya asked.

I winced.

"No. Well, that's part of it," Maya answered.

"Maybe you could wear something else?" Priya persisted.

"I don't have anything that's appropriate," Maya explained.

"App-opiate?" Anjali repeated.

"Appropriate," Maya explained. "It's a big word. It means, the right thing to do."

"App-opiate," Anjali repeated, mouthing the word with interest.

"Close enough. Anyway, I don't know if I will really like her clothes or not. I usually don't like to wear someone else's clothes, but she was just so nice on the phone, I couldn't say no," Maya smiled.

"And her husband has some medical problems and wanted me to do a home visit, so this way I can do some medical work and Mom can meet Mrs. Rutherford," I added.

"You still have to do home visits?" Priya asked.

"Yes, at least for the next few days. We have a hospital meeting coming up in two weeks and, hopefully, that will fix everything," I said.

"Are you in trouble?" Priya asked.

I looked at Maya.

"I hope not," I said. "I think I can explain everything."

"You didn't do *anything* wrong?" Priya persisted.

"No."

"Really?"

"Yes."

"Really sure?"

"Yes."

"You won't go to jail?"

"No."

Priya thought it over. Then she turned back to Maya.

"So she's just going to *give* you her clothes because Dad can't buy them?" Priya asked.

"No, Priya, it's not like that. Everything's okay," Maya reassured her.

I slowed and made a left turn onto a country road. The Corolla bounced and there was a burst of dust and noise.

"I *want* to pay her," I said, over the din. "I know she's being nice, I just don't want to take her things without paying. We don't even know her. She knows the Templars and *they* told her that Mom was looking for something to wear to the Ball."

Maya looked outside. We were on a narrow dirt road with barbed wire fences on both sides. The road dipped and turned.

The scrub gave way to bare rock.

"Are you sure you know how to get there?" she asked.

"She gave me clear instructions," I said, "and I'm following them closely. We should be coming to a paved road soon."

The road dipped down, between two stone cliffs twenty feet tall.

"She said that the rocks are like a natural wall around her house," I recalled.

We drove on, peering. A paved road emerged to the right. There was a gate with an R on it. I went out, opened the gate, drove past, and closed it behind us.

"Did you see that little bridge there, made of tubes with spaces in between?" I pointed out. "That's called a cattle guard."

No one responded. They were looking outside, captivated.

"So pretty!" Anjali said.

There were spidery mesquites and yellow-green live oaks, and clusters of barrel cacti tall as telephone poles on either side of the road. The craggy land rolled away to a forest of live oaks. Black cattle moved along slowly in the clearings, inspecting the grass, and staring back at us. A jackrabbit darted across the road, to the girls' delight.

"I see a sign," Maya announced. "It looks like a big R."

"Sounds right," I said. "Rutherford Ranch."

I slowed down to avoid spiny Turk's head cacti and maneuvered carefully. There was increasing vegetation and the road was soon gripped by tall grasses and prickly pears and swatted by tree limbs. We went up a short incline and suddenly everything fell away. The road crested the top of a hill and we looked down into a small valley. There was an L-shaped ranch house, made of stone and wood, with big bay windows and a metal roof. The L shape framed a rectangular parking lot of gravel and caliche. There was a halo of trim ryegrass about ten feet wide around the house with clumps of red-tipped photinias and white climbing roses, some of which clambered across the front wall and stretched over the door. I drove close to the edge of the road and paused. We looked down; away from the house the valley fell away abruptly and polygonal copper and maroon wheat fields terraced the slopes.

"It's *so* beautiful!" Maya repeated.

"I love it!" Priya said, gripping the window. Anjali nodded vigorously, peering over her sister's shoulder.

"England was beautiful, too. But Texas has a different kind of beauty," Maya said. "The beauty of rocks and cacti and wide-open spaces. And *huge* blue skies!"

I parked by the front door. I picked up my briefcase and we walked to the edge and looked down again.

Mrs. Rutherford came out to greet us. She was a small, energetic lady with short white hair in tight curls. She wore a white shirt and denim jeans and sported a red bandana around her neck. She shook hands vigorously.

"It's very nice to meet you, Mrs. Rutherford," I said. "This is my wife, Maya, and these are my daughters, Priya and Anjali."

"Please call me Patty, short for Patricia," she said, shaking hands with the girls. "My husband, Robbie, is inside. He's resting. Thank you so much for coming!"

"You have a beautiful ranch," Maya commented. Patty beamed.

"Thanks for helping Maya get outfitted for the Cattlewomen's Ball," I added.

"Thank *you*," Patty said, smiling. "I thought it was rather forward of me to suggest clothes for your wife, Doctor, but I have some nice things and I wanted you to at least see them. You're about my size, my dear! Don't be shy. If you don't like my selection, well, at least you got to see our home."

Mrs. Rutherford took Maya's hand. Maya looked comfortable and happy.

"Come in, come in," she said.

The smell of baking and chocolate hit us immediately.

"I made brownies for the girls!" Patty announced. "Come into the kitchen. I haven't made brownies in so long."

"Do you have any children?" Priya asked.

Patty stopped and thought.

"No," she said, awkwardly.

"Such a big house!" Priya declared.

"We have five dogs, eight cats and three hundred head of cattle," Patty said, "so we stay pretty busy!"

"Do you have a horse?" Priya asked.

"Yes, we have eight," Patty smiled. "Would you like to ride one?"

"Yes!" Priya's eyes lit up. Anjali nodded happily.

"I feel we're imposing," I said. "You may have other things to do this afternoon."

"Not at all. This is a pleasure, having company. Agatha Templar told me that Maya is about my size, and so she is, and there's no sense in buying a wardrobe in a hurry," Patty said. "And when I heard that you're making house calls, then I had an ulterior motive."

I raised my briefcase.

"I'm here to see your husband, Robert Rutherford, for a home visit," I said.

She nodded and sat us down at the table. She had set the table for us and took out brownies from the oven and set them in the middle. She poured milk for the girls and iced tea for us. She sipped her tea for a minute, then set it aside. She watched Priya and Anjali demolish their brownies and gulp down the milk. She glanced at the wall clock.

"Let's go to the living room," she said, getting up. "I have the jackets and boots there. You can bring your tea."

We followed her hastily.

"I'm sorry if I'm rushing you. Robbie, my husband, will need his afternoon medicines soon. Normally, he has lunch and then takes his medicines himself but today he didn't and I have to give them to him."

We were ushered into a large living room with black leather sofas, a rocking chair draped with cowhide and several rough-hewn wooden chairs arranged around a glass coffee table made of antlers.

"Make yourselves comfortable, please," Patty said. "I'll be right back. I'm going to give Robbie his medicines. I'll get you the jackets. The shoes are right there, Maya, behind the ottoman. Try them on till then."

She left in a hurry.

We did not sit down. We walked around the room slowly. Anjali and Priya held hands as they explored. The room had brown shag carpet and smelled of cigar smoke and leather polish. The walls were bottle green and there were dark squares and rectangles at eye level but no pictures or framed art.

Maya and I moved to a large bay window which looked out on the valley below. The girls ventured into a study. They froze when they saw a mounted stag's head. They discovered two more and three boars' heads and a stuffed bobcat next to a desk. They shot back to Maya and huddled next to her.

"I don't like this place," Priya said. "It's scary!"

Anjali scowled and grasped Maya's skirt.

"Some people like to hunt," Maya explained.

"I don't like killing things," Priya retorted.

"Different people have different thoughts," Maya said.

We waited silently by the bay window. I heard voices in the

other room, Patty's and a man's voice.

"No, I won't!" the man said loudly.

Mrs. Rutherford said something unintelligible.

"No, I *won't!*" the man repeated, angrily.

There was a rustling, and Patty came out, holding a tan leather jacket in a hanger with a plastic cover, and a pair of matching boots. She shook her head and looked down. She set the boots down and looked back.

"Foreigner! Wetback!" the man's voice rang out.

Patty flushed.

"I really wanted you to meet Robbie, Doctor, and give him some advice, medical advice, you know," she explained, "but my Robbie is in one of his moods. I'm sorry for his behavior."

She held up the jacket and rotated it, showing the layers criss-crossing the front and back, creating intricate details, with tassels trimming the outer margins. Maya was impressed.

"I bought it in Vegas, at the National Rodeo," Patty smiled. "Actually, Robbie bought it for me. At an auction. I have the same set in red, but I thought the tan would look so good on you, my dear. Can you believe, I never wore it!"

"Why not?" Maya asked.

Patty shrugged and looked away.

"Oh, this thing and that," she answered, after a short pause. "Anyway, it's never been worn. Robbie also bought these boots for me and they match the jacket. I can tell that we have the same size, but try them on. You wear size six shoes? Or six and a half?"

"Six," Maya said.

"And the jacket is petite," Patty said, and helped Maya try it on. It fit well.

"Not perfect, but pretty good," Patty said. "Luckily you're so pretty that no one will ever notice the jacket!"

Maya blushed and protested.

"Now the boots."

The boots were tight in the front, but Patty insisted we take them.

"Just wear them at home for a few days, they'll open up."

"I'll return them right after the ball," Maya promised.

"Keep them as long as you want," Patty said, and stepped back to see Maya in the jacket and boots. She clapped her hands in the air excitedly.

"Oh, you look *so* good!" she declared. "You'll fit right in. You'll be the belle of the ball!"

"Thank you so much," Maya said. Priya and Anjali nodded enthusiastically.

"Get ready to do the two-step!" Patty said. "There's going to be lots of dancing!"

"Patt-tee!" Robbie's voice boomed. He sounded angrier.

Patty picked up Maya's shoes and handed them to her.

"Keep wearing the boots, my dear, let them open up. Robbie needs me," she said, ushering us out. "I have to go. Thank you so much for coming. Doctor, would you mind if I call you later?"

"Feel free," I said. "I can come back to do a house call at another time, if Mr. Rutherford wants."

"Bless your heart, you're patient," she sighed. "Robbie doesn't want to see you right now, but I'm going to have Tommy Templar talk to him."

"Patt-tee! Patt-*tee!*" Robbie screamed. Patty turned and ran back. Maya picked up the jacket and her shoes and we prepared to leave.

Patty reappeared, flustered.

"Doctor, I'm so sorry about Robbie. He just talked to Tommy and he's changed his mind. Now, he does want to see you. Will you see him? Will you do a home visit right now?"

"Sure. I need to confirm, is he disabled?"

"Yes, he has diabetes and hasn't been out of the house in a very long time."

"For Medicare rules, I have to check that he has been home bound for the last twelve weeks or so," I explained.

"He's been home bound for much longer than that," Patty answered quickly.

I glanced at Maya. She nodded.

"I'll have my lady ranch hand Tammy Sue take Maya and the girls and show them the horses," Patty said, "and I will introduce you to my husband. Let me warn you: he's not in a good mood."

After Tammy Sue appeared and escorted the girls away, I followed Patty through a short passageway to a large gloomy bedroom facing east. The room was darker and cooler and smelled strongly of cigars and stale linen. It had the same brown shag carpet and the walls were lined with dark wood panels. A low bed on the left faced a large window on the right. The long wall facing me was adorned with mounted heads of stags and bison.

Mr. Rutherford sat up in bed. He was a huge man, over three hundred and fifty pounds, with a large red face and bulbous eyes. He looked like a giant amoeba oozing out of blue pajamas. He peered at me through thick glasses as I entered and adjusted his oxygen tubing. He wheezed as he spoke.

"Doctor, come here!" he commanded. "Sit you down right here, where I can see you."

I sat down close to him. He peered at me keenly.

"Mexican?" he asked.

"No," I replied, "Indian."

"Same thing," he said and shook his head. He looked out the large window. I was determined to remain calm so I gazed out the window as well and waited for him to speak.

"Indian!" he repeated. "Where's the damned Americans?"

The window was framed by climbing roses and looked out onto a rocky slope sporting withered brown lantana and blackened Turk's Caps.

I listened to him breathe for a few minutes but said nothing.

"I like that, that you don't talk too much," he said, without turning.

I said nothing, pressing my advantage.

"You like plants, *Mr.* Mather?" he asked.

"Yes," I answered.

"Do you see the lantana and the Turk's Caps?"

"Yes," I said, careful not to say *sir*.

"You know, I planted them myself. Know why?"

I paused.

"Because they come back every year," I guessed.

"Exactly!" he rubbed his hands. "Because they come back every year. And they get better and better every year. The yellow lantana, it's hardy. Not the red. Not the white. Not the pink. Only the yellow."

I grunted.

"You know why the other one's called Turk's Caps?"

"Yes."

He turned to me.

"Why?" he asked.

"Because the small red flowers look like the red caps that Turkish people wear," I answered. "But it's in the same family as the Hibiscus, or shoe flower."

Robbie looked in front.

"Maybe you aren't completely dull, Mr. Mathur," he said. "You hunt?"

"No."

He looked victorious.

"Hah! Thought so!" he crowed.

"Mr. Rutherford, your wife said you had some medical problems. What are they?" I asked bluntly.

"Oh, come now, come now, don't be so irritated, little man," he said, happily. "I can tell you're irritated!"

I said nothing and looked out the window.

"I'm seventy. I have diabetes and high blood pressure. Two heart attacks, so they say. Felt nothing, nothing at all. I reckon it was on account of the diabetes, because it gives you silent heart attacks. No cancer. Gained weight and got diabetes on account of that, and I refuse to take insulin. Yes, sir, I refuse. No shots. Take pills for diabetes and pressure. *Patt-tee!* Patty'll show you."

Patty appeared with two bottles. I switched the table lamp on and read the labels.

"You're on metformin 500 mg twice daily for diabetes and lisinopril 5 mg daily for blood pressure control," I read.

"Look-ee mama!" he said to Patty, "the little Indian doctor can read English!"

Patty and I glared at him. He chuckled.

"So what's the problem?" I asked, again.

He sighed and raised his hands and tugged back the sleeves. He had fingers like sausages and hands like balloons.

"Look at my fingers and arms! I got a rash, little man!" he said.

I ignored his taunts. I swung the bedside lamp to get a better look. He had several red patches on his wrists and his fingers with raised edges and flat centers and scaling. The skin in between was inflamed.

"What have you been using?" I asked.

"How do you know I've been using anything?" he asked, surprised.

"You have a rash, but the skin in-between is also red and inflamed. That usually happens when you use a steroid cream."

"You're right, little man," he said, his tone a little softer. "Mama, show him that cream."

Patty looked on a shelf and extracted a tube.

"Triamcinolone 0.01%" I read. "That's a potent steroid!"

"You mean, it's strong?" Robbie asked.

"Yes. Did it make the rash better or worse?"

Robbie shrugged.

"Worse," said Patty.

"You have five dogs and eight cats, right?" I asked.

"Yes, little man," he said. "I bet Patty told you that."

"Do you have this rash anywhere else on your body?" I asked, determined to ignore Robbie's sarcastic tone.

"Yeah!" Robbie answered and lifted up his pajama shirt and eased his shorts down a little. There were a few patches in his groins. Again, they were about an inch in diameter with raised edges and flat centers and scaling.

"Got worse with steroids?" I asked again.

"Yeah," Robbie said, and covered up. He glared at Patty.

I thought of the possibilities. I was silent for a minute.

"Guess we wasted our time!" Robbie remarked, bitterly. "The man has no clue. That Tommy better be more careful with his recommendations!"

"I think you have a yeast infection on your skin," I said cautiously.

"Why would I get a skin infection? Robbie asked, derisively, "when my wife bathes me every day? Eh?"

"You have dogs and they lie in bed with you."

"Patty told you?"

"No, I see dog hair on your sheets and pajamas. You're diabetic, so you're prone to infections and you may not even feel them very much, because you have nerve damage so you don't feel the pain."

"Really?" he sounded doubtful.

"You just said you didn't feel your heart attacks, due to the diabetes damaging your nerves," I said.

He looked at me in surprise and confusion.

"You *really* think it's a fungal infection?" he asked.

"Yes," I said. "I've seen several. You are diabetic, that's a big risk factor. Do you have good control of your diabetes?"

"Sometimes," he admitted. Patty shook her head grimly.

"Stop the steroid cream, the one you borrowed from your wife," I insisted. "Apply some anti-fungal cream and stay away from your pets in the evening."

"What should I use? Can you write me a prescription?"

"Just get some athlete's foot cream. It is much cheaper than prescription anti-fungal ointments. Just as good."

"I can do that."

"And I'm going to guess that you have a hard time drying and cleaning your toes," I added.

"Look at me, little man!" Robbie burst out. "I can't even see my toes!"

"Dry your feet with a hair dryer. The space between the toes is where yeast infection starts," I advised.

Robbie looked at his feet and nodded.

"Doc, I need to save money. I can't work on account of my knees and my back."

"Right. So save money by buying over-the-counter ointment for athlete's foot. It's a great antifungal. Apply it twice daily for two months, night and day, and keep your feet really dry. Use a hair dryer to dry your feet."

"Okay!" Robbie agreed, reluctantly.

"Let me examine you," I said, and he nodded. I examined his

puffy hands and checked his pulse. I checked his blood pressure and listened to his chest and noted wheezing in both lungs. His abdomen was protuberant and the same rash was florid in his groins. He wouldn't let me examine deeper. His legs were swollen and had weak pulses. His feet were numb. I checked his reflexes. They were intact. I removed his glasses and saw that his left eyelid was drooping and the left eye looked downwards and outwards.

"Do you have double vision?" I asked.

"Yes, when I look to the right."

"You never told me that!" Patty burst out.

Robbie shrugged.

I shone a flashlight in both eyes. I made him follow the tip of my finger with his eyes as I moved my finger in the outline of a cross.

"Your pupils respond to light. That's good. But your left eye does not turn completely to the right. Do you have any pain in your eyes?"

"I did, months ago."

Patty shook her head in disbelief.

"You have diabetic nerve damage of the left third cranial nerve, the one that works the little muscles of the eye. You also have diabetic nerve damage in your legs, causing numbness in your feet."

Patty was shocked.

"What should we do?" she asked.

"Did you get a CT or MRI of the head, just to be sure there wasn't an aneurysm or something else pressing on the third cranial nerve?"

Robbie nodded his head.

"Went to a specialist in Fort Worth. He ran all kinds of tests, CT, MRI, you name it. What's your best guess, little man?"

"Usually, if the pupil is spared, as it is in your case, then it's due to diabetes, so that's my best guess. I bet the tests were all normal, no aneurysm."

Robbie grunted.

"And my legs?" he asked.

"There's loss of sensation in your legs but you still have your reflexes. That's typical."

He stared at me.

"I don't understand how you know that the weakness in my eye is because of diabetes and not something like an aneurysm," he growled. "The specialists in Fort Worth were confused."

"Think of it like your TV. The video and cable wires run up behind it side by side. If you can't play a video but you still get cable, then there's probably something wrong with the video player, or it's just not turned on, or something like that. But if you aren't getting a cable signal or a video signal then it's unlikely that both the video player and the cable box have broken down; it's more likely that both video and cable wires are messed up where they run together."

"So what you're saying is, an aneurysm or tumor would eat into both wires, not just one?"

"Exactly."

Mr. Rutherford shook his head and nodded.

"I went to Dallas. Didn't tell Patty. Spent five thousand bucks. MRI was good. Said the exact same thing. No tumor, no aneurysm. Darn it! Gosh darn it!"

He laughed.

"And here you are, figuring the same thing, in my bedroom in the corner of Hotspur County!" he said, bitterly. His shoulders sagged, "Wasted five thousand dollars!"

"I would have probably ordered those tests, too, just to be sure," I said.

Robbie stared at me.

"Maybe you're okay," he admitted. "Maybe you're not just full of it, like a lot of the doctors I see these days. Just want to do a wallet biopsy, most of them."

He pulled up his blanket and lay down. I got up.

"If you use the cream, you should be better in ten days. Is there anything else?"

Robbie looked away.

"One more thing. Tell me, your parents living?" he asked.

"Yes."

"In India?"

"Yes."

"Must be proud of you?"

I was puzzled.

"Sometimes," I answered.

He laughed bitterly.

"Wish I had a son I was proud of," he said. He stopped himself and rummaged in the blanket for the remote control.

"Wish I had a son," he said, and glared at Patty. Patty looked away.

Mr. Rutherford found the remote and studied it.

"I don't have a son. No son!" He looked away. "You have a son?"

"No. Two daughters."

He nodded.

"What does your father do?"

"He's a professor in a medical school."

"And your mother?"

"She's a pathologist."

"Two doctors? How did that happen?"

"They met in medical school."

"They wanted you to be a doctor?"

"No. Anything but a doctor."

"Anything but a doctor! Why?"

"They had seen the rough side of medicine. The long years of studying, the hours of being on call and away from family, rushing off for emergencies."

"Getting fired from your hospital and forced to make house calls on painful rednecks?"

I smiled.

"Never a dull moment," I said.

Mr. Rutherford chuckled.

"I wanted to see what kind of guy you were," he explained. "You're okay. You can go now. My show's fixing to start."

Patty walked me out. Robbie turned on the TV.

"Does he have that rash in his private areas?" I asked Patty.

"Yes. How did you know that?" she asked.

"It's a favorite spot for yeast infections in diabetics. Keep his skin very dry, especially after you bathe him," I advised. "Especially as he doesn't seem too concerned about his health."

"Don't be upset, Doctor," she said. "He treats everyone like this, even Tommy."

"Even Tommy Templar?"

"They went to school together, Hotspur High, class of '42," Patty said.

"We're having them over for dinner next weekend," I said. "They've kind of adopted us. They're wonderful."

"They've been bragging on you. Tommy told Robbie to have you do a home visit, and he did."

"Tommy needs to tell him to stop smoking cigars," I said.

She shook her head.

"He won't listen to anyone about that!"

"Smoking is a big risk, and he's overweight, has high cholesterol and diabetes. This is a terrible place to have a heart attack!"

Patty froze, struck by the thought.

"Maybe you should come back sometime, in a couple of weeks, for a follow-up visit."

"Let's see how he does," I dodged. "His regular doctor is Dr. Becker, right? Dr. Becker will be back soon."

"Karl doesn't like to make home visits," Patty said.

"I plan to write a note about my visit and send it to Dr. Becker. Would you like a copy?"

"Yes, Doctor," Patty said.

I checked to make sure I had my stethoscope, blood pressure apparatus, torch, and knee hammer. I revised my note mentally and reviewed Robbie's allergies and family history. I scribbled points for dictation and thanked Patty.

Tammy Sue and the girls were outside in the parking area, petting a gray mare.

"I loved the horses!" Priya gushed, "and she gave us the brownies to take home!"

"I love the jacket!" Maya declared. "I'm going to buy one just like it!"

"Love it!" Anjali chimed, beaming.

Patty nuzzled the mare and Tammy Sue waved goodbye.

We wove past the rocky cliffs and down the paved road to the cattle guard and closed the gate carefully behind us. The wind had picked up and gusts of dust and leaves peppered the windscreen.

"I like Patty," I said, "but Mr. Rutherford is a little nasty."

"Don't worry about him," Maya said. "You have the big board meeting coming up. Are you ready for it?"

"Yes, I went down to medical records and reviewed the chart. I think I've found something."

Maya held up her hand.

"I think I also found something today. In the big room, did you notice those dark squares on the walls of the living room?" Maya asked. "I noticed them when you were with Mr. Rutherford."

"Yes," I said.

"Looked like some pictures were hanging there, and were removed," she said. "You think they removed some family pictures?"

"It's possible. I wonder if he had a son," I said. "He seemed bitter and said he didn't have a son. Maybe he had a son who left or maybe they didn't get along."

"I can ask Agatha about the Rutherfords. This is a small town. Everyone knows everything."

"Yes," I said, "and that's scary. There are no secrets in small towns. Everyone knows everything, eventually."

CHAPTER 8

THE BOARD MEETING

Emily Youngblood stood up and cleared her throat. The crowd grew silent.

"The Hospital Board is meeting today here in the Hotspur Hospital cafeteria to discuss a concern of Dr. Ehrlich, who is the acting chief of medical staff," she announced. "We have invited Mrs. Angela Aguilar, as a representative of the Texas Medical Board, from Austin."

A plump lady in a grey pantsuit stood up, waved, and sat down. She smiled at the gathering.

Emily Youngblood continued.

"The Hospital Board states for the public that the matter concerns the death of a resident of Hotspur County. These matters will be discussed in private, and the public is asked to vacate the cafeteria after two opening statements are made," she finished.

I sat at one of the front tables with Maya and Simon facing the board. I glanced at Dr. Ehrlich sitting at the other table. His face shone; his hair was neatly parted in the middle and he wore a dark suit and tie. He pushed back from his table and stood up stiffly. He turned to address the crowd.

"I am Dr. Ehrlich. I am a specialist in internal medicine. I daresay I know everyone in this room because I've been coming here since I graduated from the University of Texas Medical Branch in Galveston years and years ago, when a lot of you were still in diapers! Diapers! I have been coming here from the Metroplex off and on to moonlight. I have a very busy practice in Dallas but I still come back here often. Why? Because I love y'all like family. Family! Y'all are wonderful folks."

He paused. There was a polite round of applause.

"I am trusted with the medical care of this wonderful community. I take that responsibility very seriously. Very seriously! I feel there has been poor care, poor, poor care of a citizen of this county and that, sadly, contributed to his death. I asked for this meeting to be held as soon as possible so we can deliver justice! Yea, justice!"

He turned around and glared at me.

"Justice must be done! We have these foreign doctors and nurses who come here. Why are they here, I ask you? If they were so good at their jobs, why did they have to leave their own countries, eh? Ask yourselves that, my friends! I will tell you why. Because they are the rejects who couldn't make it in their own countries. What are they doing here? They take advantage of your kindness and betray your trust through their incompetence!"

I was gratified that the audience remained solidly silent. Emily Youngblood turned to Mrs. Aguilar and spoke in a stage whisper.

"Can he *say* things like that about foreign doctors and nurses?" Emily asked.

"Depends on your hospital rules," Mrs. Aguilar answered, calmly.

Emily looked at the four other board members. They were uncomfortable but shrugged.

"I have a right to express myself, Mrs. Youngblood!" Dr. Ehrlich said. "I am the only American out of the three medical staff who were in the ER that night. It's my right, I can say whatever I want."

"We will treat everyone equally," Mrs. Youngblood said firmly. "We are evaluating medical care, not citizenship. If you are done, Dr. Mathur has a statement."

"Done? I'm not done. The only way you can tell if something's *done* is to stick a knife into it," Dr. Ehrlich quipped. There was a titter in the audience.

"Would you like to say something else?" Mrs. Youngblood asked, dryly.

"Yes. I want to tell this audience not to believe a word these two say. Dr. Mathur and Simon Godwyn are in a plot to discredit me and cover up their failures. Don't believe a word they say! Their foreign training is piss-poor! Piss-poor! They caused the death of our dear friend Guillermo. We cannot allow them to stay here and risk it happening again."

He pointed at Simon and me and shook his head gravely. He sat down heavily.

I stood up and turned to face the crowd.

"Thank you for coming today. I know the hospital means a lot to all of you. It means a lot to me and my family, too. I want to state for the record that this meeting was going to be rescheduled to allow the deceased's wife to return from Mexico, as she had critical evidence, but the meeting was actually moved up rather than down. This makes it unfair as an important witness will be missing. Therefore I request that the meeting be postponed."

The board whispered amongst themselves. Dr. Ehrlich shook his head vigorously.

"The Chamber of Commerce meeting is tomorrow and Dr. Ehrlich is not available the rest of the week," Emily Youngblood explained. "I'm afraid we have to proceed."

"I may not be able to prove my case without the deceased's wife," I explained.

Dr. Ehrlich smirked.

"You *have* no case, witness or no witness," he declared.

"Ignore him, Dr. Mathur," Simon whispered.

"The meeting will continue. Dr. Ehrlich is currently our

Medical Chief. The board has agreed to his recommendations and needs to make some decisions. The board wants to review the evidence in private," Mrs. Youngblood announced. "The public is requested to leave."

There was a rattling of chairs and tables as the men and women filed out. They could be seen through the narrow windows of the cafeteria, talking to each other in the parking lot. Emily Youngblood closed the doors and returned to her seat.

"We will now get to the medical business at hand. Dr. Ehrlich will make his medical statement first and then Dr. Mathur."

Dr. Ehrlich rose majestically.

"Members of the board," he said, waving his hand at them. "Members of the board! You are entrusted with the healthcare of the citizens who elected you. It is a sacred duty! Sacred duty! I am here to guide you in that sacred duty! I must inform you that, on the night of November 17th, I was on call in the ER. I was called to see a Mr. Guillermo Guttierrez, who was brought in by ambulance. He had been found collapsed at home by his wife. We do not know how much time he had been unconscious before he was discovered by his family."

He pointed to me.

"This doctor was not on call. This male nurse, sitting next to him, called him without my consent. Without my consent! This nurse is from England but obviously doesn't understand English!"

Simon bit his lip but said nothing.

"This doctor came and made not one but two fatal mistakes! Mistakes that caused the patient to die that night!"

Mrs. Aguilar sat up straight and listened intently.

"There were two mistakes: he delivered an electric shock so badly, that the patient's chest set on fire, and he gave a lethal dose of potassium to the patient, even though the potassium was normal."

Maya turned to look at me.

"You said *he* gave the shock," she asked.

"He did! He's lying!" I answered.

"Why would he lie?" she asked again.

"I bet he's embarrassed about it," I whispered.

Simon rummaged through his briefcase and pulled out a large white FedEx envelope.

"Dr. Ehrlich, both Dr. Mathur and the nurse Simon Godwyn have stated that you were the one who gave the shock that caused the burning," Mrs. Youngblood said.

"They're lying! You can't believe them! Dr. Mathur is lying because he wants to get his green card and doesn't want anything that would look bad on his application. He's so desperate that he even brought along his wife to get your sympathy. Simon is also a foreigner and married a Hotspur girl just to get a green card!"

Simon turned red with anger and snorted. The board looked at me and then at Simon.

Simon stood up.

"May I say something, Your Honors?" he said, smoothly but coldly.

The board was taken aback.

"You don't have to call us Your Honors," Mrs. Youngblood said. "This isn't England!"

"Be that as it may, I would just as soon maintain decorum. And I further would request your indulgence to address your honorable selves with the greatest of deference."

The board was confused.

"What, exactly, do you mean, Simon?" Emily Youngblood asked.

"May I proceed?" Simon asked, with such urbane

smoothness that the board nodded in unison.

"I have reviewed the laws that are applicable to this matter and must state for the august board present herein, that there was a third witness to the event of the conflagration of the unfortunate patient!"

"What?" Dr. Ehrlich burst out. "Another witness? Impossible!"

"Nevertheless, it is true," Simon said, and struck a dramatic pose. I was flabbergasted and sat down. Simon was the star and I was eclipsed.

The board members gagged and looked at Mrs. Aguilar.

"Who is this third witness?" she demanded. "There were only the three of you in the room!"

Simon brandished a large FedEx envelope and glanced inside.

"The man's wife. She was standing right outside the door," Simon answered.

"Impossible! I closed the door!" Dr. Ehrlich cried.

"Yes, but the door would not stay closed, Dr. Ehrlich. You remember you pushed the stool against it? It never closed completely, unfortunately."

"Now I remember! She told me in David Dawkins' office that she saw you set him on fire! She thought you were just doing everything possible!" I burst out.

"Ridiculous!"Ced Dr. Ehrlich dismissed.

"Let's get her testimony!" I pleaded.

"So where is she, this amazing witness?" Dr. Ehrlich demanded.

"She is in Mexico, where she ought to be, attending to the final wishes of her husband and settling family affairs," Simon said.

"So there is no witness at this meeting now!" Dr. Ehrlich

crowed.

"Dr. Ehrlich, do you deny that *you* and *not* Dr. Mathur delivered the ill-fated shock that set the unfortunate man's chest on fire?" Simon asked, and approached Dr. Ehrlich's table.

"Of course I deny it!"

"Do you swear to it?" Simon demanded, his voice rising.

"Yes, I do!" Dr. Ehrlich stood up and glared back at Simon.

Simon returned to our table and picked up the FedEx envelope.

"What would you say if I said I had a signed, certified statement from the wife that she spoke to you after the event and she saw *you* deliver that shock, and she thanked you for everything and that you *admitted* to her that *you* had delivered that shock?"

Dr. Ehrlich stood, his mouth open, and said nothing.

"Would you still swear it was not you? Under oath? Risking your medical license?" Simon asked, waving the white envelope.

Dr. Ehrlich swallowed. He looked at the board, helplessly. The board members looked at each other, confused.

"Would you like me to unseal this envelope and deliver the contents to Mrs. Aguilar and the Texas State Medical Board," Simon demanded.

Dr. Ehrlich opened his mouth but said nothing.

"Dr. Ehrlich, would you like to just withdraw this matter of the chest setting on fire?" Mrs. Youngblood asked, quietly.

Dr. Ehrlich scowled.

Simon approached the board members with the envelope.

"Stop!" Dr Ehrlich barked.

Simon looked at him impassively. Dr. Ehrlich's face contorted.

"Yes!" he snapped. "I withdraw that matter!"

A sigh of relief swept the room. Simon nodded and sat

down. He turned and winked. Dr. Ehrlich was livid.

"But I still press my other charge about the potassium! That was the mistake that killed the man! That was the fatal mistake! Explain that!" Dr. Ehrlich shrieked.

I stood up.

"May I explain?" I asked.

Mrs. Youngblood nodded.

"In our lab, the normal potassium is three point one to four point eight, and the patient's potassium was three point zero. So it was already a little low. But the way that sample was obtained, I'm sure the sample was traumatized and the red blood cells were squeezed so some potassium leaked out of them. That meant the low reading was wrong, and the correct value was much lower."

"What do you mean by a traumatized sample?" Henry Odell, a Board member, asked.

"The sample was drawn with difficulty, from three different sites, with a great deal of suctioning, or pulling back, to get the blood sample," I explained. "That caused the red blood cells to break down. They have lots of potassium inside. The potassium that leaks out gives a falsely high reading of potassium on the sample."

"Not true!" Dr. Ehrlich declared. "That sample was obtained without any problems."

"I dispute that," I countered. "And you can see from the autopsy report that there were twelve needle marks on his arms and legs. Multiple attempts, because of multiple failures."

"The failed attempts were by the paramedics!" Dr. Ehrlich declared.

"No, they were not," I rebutted. "I looked at the paramedics' records. Only two tries, the second one was successful. It's all there if you want to read it."

I placed the papers on Dr. Ehrlich's desk. He pushed them

away.

"I don't want to read it! All that matters is that the potassium was normal and you pushed more potassium," he retorted.

"The patient was also taking diuretics, medicines that make you pass a lot of urine," I explained. "He was taking a powerful diuretic called metolazone. It's notorious for causing a very low potassium."

"We only have one potassium result!" Dr. Ehrlich yelled. "Stop this nonsense! We have just one result!"

I thought for a minute. I played my ace.

"Actually, we may be able to get another potassium level," I said, quietly.

"Ridiculous!" Dr. Ehrlich declared.

Mrs. Aguilar spoke up.

"I need to say something," she said.

The board nodded.

"I am an RN, and I used to work in an ICU. For me, a potassium of three point zero is low. Not normal, but low. I think there is a rationale for giving potassium."

"Ridiculous!" Dr. Ehrlich repeated, a little less loudly.

"If we somehow recheck the potassium, and I don't know how we could run the same sample again, but *if* we could somehow check it again and find the correct value, and *if* it were low, lower than three point zero, then Dr. Mathur and this Hospital Board could potentially make a case against *Dr. Ehrlich* for *not* giving the potassium!" she explained.

Dr. Ehrlich was shocked.

"How dare you!" he exploded.

"I'm merely stating my opinion," Mrs. Aguilar answered, coolly.

Dr. Ehrlich stood up and pointed at Mrs. Aguilar.

"How dare you talk to me like that!" he screamed. He

scrambled out of his chair and stood in front of Mrs. Aguilar and glared at her. "How dare you?"

"Sit down! Sit down, Dr. Ehrlich!" Mrs. Youngblood pounded her desk.

Eventually, Dr. Ehrlich sat down.

"How are we going to get another potassium level?" Mrs. Youngblood asked me.

"I remembered that we drew an arterial blood sample for the blood gases. The sample was frozen, along with the venous sample that had been checked. Why not thaw out the arterial blood sample and run a potassium on it? It was obtained without difficulty," I said.

"Is that reasonable, Dr. Ehrlich?" Mrs. Youngblood asked.

"I don't care," he responded.

"You do understand what Mrs. Aguilar just said, don't you?" Mrs. Youngblood persisted.

Dr. Ehrlich hesitated.

"Yes," he admitted.

"Do you want to go ahead and check the potassium in the frozen arterial sample, or should we just drop this matter as well?" she asked, pointedly. "Dr. Mathur is certainly risking his green card and his license, but you may be jeopardizing your considerable reputation here."

"Maybe even *your* license," Mrs. Aguilar added.

All eyes were on Dr. Ehrlich.

"Do it! Damn it all, do it! Check the potassium in the damn arterial sample!" Dr. Ehrlich snapped. "Damn foreigners telling us how to practice medicine! Do it!"

Mrs. Youngblood looked at Mrs. Aguilar and shrugged.

"I will go to Tom Lightfoot in the lab and tell him to run the frozen arterial sample," she said, and excused herself.

Thirty agonizing minutes went by. Maya had left the girls with Mrs. Marsh, because Billie Priestley, our usual sitter, wanted to attend the meeting. Maya called to check on them. I recalled my experience with patients on metolazone. I remembered they often had dangerously low potassium levels. I remembered Mr. Guttierrez's EKG. It had shown features of a low potassium, the low T waves and the sagging ST segments. That almost always happened at potassium levels below three point zero. But then there was the blood report of a level of three point zero. Something did not fit; that happened all the time in medicine, *something* just would not fit.

I turned to Simon.

"How were you able to get that statement from Mrs. Gutierrez?" I asked quietly.

He grinned and bowed his head.

"What statement, Doctor?" he said.

"The one in that FedEx envelope!"

"I never said there was a statement from her in that envelope," he whispered.

"You said you had a statement from her!"

Simon shook his head.

"No, I merely asked the august gentleman what he would say *if* I had a statement from Mrs. G," he whispered. "I never said I *had* the statement."

I recoiled in surprise.

"I'm sorry, was that statement subject to misinterpretation?" Simon asked, smiling innocently.

I was at a loss.

"Subject to misinterpretation?" I gagged. "You *lied!*"

"I wasn't lying, I was being economical with the truth, Doctor," Simon replied, and looked at me blankly. "Merely economical with the truth."

I had to suppress a guffaw.

Emily Youngblood returned with Tom Lightfoot, the lab director. She looked at Dr. Ehrlich.

"Do you want us to proceed or should we drop this matter right now?" she asked him, sharply.

"Go ahead!" he snapped. "Do your damnedest!"

"Very well. Tom will read the result. We ran it three times, just to be sure, and we're sorry for the delay."

Tom spoke in his gravelly monotone.

"The arterial blood sample from deceased patient Gutierrez, obtained eleven-seventeen of nineteen ninety-six, showed a potassium of two point seven," he announced.

I hugged Maya. Simon slapped me on the back.

"Bloody good show!" he roared. "*Bloody brilliant!*"

After the excitement died down, Mrs. Youngblood spoke.

"Dr. Mathur, you are reinstated. As our new Chief of Medical Staff, do you wish to pursue action against Dr. Ehrlich?"

Before I could answer, Mrs. Aguilar interrupted.

"Hold on! Now the State Board has an interest in this matter. This matter should be put off until review by TMB in Austin. We must end it here for tonight. We need to obtain legal opinions. Dr. Ehrlich, I advise you to obtain legal advice as well."

I was happy with that. We rushed to pack up, desperate to go home and tell Priya and Anjali the good news. I could have cried with relief.

Dr. Ehrlich stormed out of the room, slamming the doors as he left.

Mrs. Aguilar handed me a printed statement.

"This states that all charges are dropped and you acted in keeping with best practices of medicine," she smiled. "Keep it carefully. You will need it for your green card interview."

I glanced at the document as she walked away.

Simon cleared his throat.

"I just *happen* to have a completely empty FedEx envelope you can put that in," he drawled.

CHAPTER 9

THE LAST HOME VISIT

I knotted my tie and slid it up into place.

"I think this is going to be my last home visit," I said.

"Do you have a nice jacket to go with that tie?" Maya asked.

"I have that tweed jacket from London."

"The tweed jacket? No. It looks like you're wearing a blanket. Wear the new brown coat you bought in Houston for job interviews. Remember, you have to come for the Chamber of Commerce lunch after you see your patient. By the way, your patient, Mr. Woodcox, used to be the mayor."

"Actually, his wife is the patient. Yes, Mr. Woodcox used to be the mayor," I said, "but he resigned."

"Never mind, wear the new brown jacket." Maya advised.

"It's not waterproof," I protested

"There's no rain in the forecast."

"Wind advisory," I said. "They're predicting a big sand storm called a haboob. There was a huge storm in Jarrell, over twenty people died."

But Maya insisted, so I selected the brown jacket. I admit, it looked neat. Maya came up to inspect.

"That looks more presentable," she said.

"That sounds like an architect," I replied.

I tied my shoes and stood up.

"I'll see you at the Chamber at lunch. Where will the girls stay?"

"Right here at home. Billie Priestley is coming over to babysit. You remember sweet Billie?" Maya said.

I grinned.

"Oh, yes! She helped us unpack the day we moved here from Houston and at 9 p.m., when you and I were dead tired, she said she was going dancing!"

"She's in her seventies but she's full of energy," Maya said. "And she still goes dancing every Saturday!"

"Maybe we should go dancing too," I said. "I don't know how to dance, but how hard can it be?"

The air was gritty and the sky was the color of wet sand. The Corolla was covered with a layer of dust. I wiped down the windows and drove down the hill. I turned left on Commercial, drove four blocks and turned right on Walnut. The Woodcox residence occupied an entire block. I parked on the road and stopped myself applying the steering wheel lock, an old habit from Houston. I reached for the mouthwash instead.

The lot was screened by mature live oak and pecan trees, lined up neatly behind the sidewalk. The gate had been left open. I walked in and closed it carefully. The house was a handsome, two-story residence with white brick walls and decorated columns. The front door was approached by a set of steps and was framed by two large planters. I stood in front of the door and looked around. The front lawn was unkempt. The grass had withered and large parts were bare. Flowering mustard weeds and dandelions flourished in some of the bald patches. Close to the house, there were dried pansies and blackened lantana. The planters had once held English Ivy and ornamental grass; dried remnants hung over the edges and crunched underfoot.

The door opened and a short man with thin white hair greeted me. He wore a crisp white shirt and pressed jeans.

"Hey! Dr. Mathur!" he said, warmly. "Willis Woodcox! Come on in!"

We shook hands. He took my jacket and hung it on a metal

coat stand that looked like a drilling tower.

"Come on inside! Can I get you anything to drink? Tea? Coffee?" he asked.

"I'm fine, thank you."

"Sit down and make yourself comfortable. Sarah will be right here. She's getting ready for the Chamber lunch. It's always been such a big deal for her. She used to be the secretary of the Chamber, you know!" he said.

I sat down on a sofa and looked around. The room was dark. The window was shrouded by thick blue curtains and the walls were covered with yellow crepe wallpaper. Four high back chairs were arranged around the sofa and a coffee table in front had an assortment of pill bottles and a folder. Two floor lamps near the doors provided a little light. I expected my host to pull the curtains back.

"Tommy and Agatha Templar recommended you highly, Dr. Mathur! Normally, we go to Dallas to see specialists there, but we would much rather keep our business in town. I'm a retired oilman, might say I never really retired. Friends everywhere, so Dallas is like a second home. You been to Dallas, Doc?"

"A few times," I said.

"Sarah's been going there, sees specialists there for her nerves - neuropathy, I mean - and such."

"Mr. Woodcox, are these Sarah's medicines?" I asked, pointing to the coffee table.

"Yes, and that's her file. Go ahead, you can read it."

I picked up the bottles and the file but couldn't read them in the dark. I stood up and walked to the table lamp.

"Let me open the curtains a little," Mr. Woodcox said.

"Leave them closed!" a sharp voice snapped.

Mrs. Woodcox appeared. She was a tall, slender lady wearing a knee-length black dress, long black gloves and a small black hat. She held a clutch in her left hand and offered her right. We shook and we sat down. She stared at me.

"I would like you to fill my medications," she announced. "That's all."

"Of course. But this is the first time I've met you. I need to take a history and examine you."

"No!" she was vehement. "Just refill the medicines!"

"Darling, he can't just give you medicines without seeing you," Mr. Woodcox explained.

"No!" she repeated. "I said no!"

"I need to talk to you and examine you. I will be brief, I promise," I said.

"No! Write my prescriptions and leave!" she repeated.

I looked at her husband. He moved to her side and kneeled and spoke softly with his face looking up to hers.

"Darling, he's just doing what a doctor has to do. He has to talk to you and examine you. That's the law," he explained.

"No! I already have specialists! I don't need another quack!" she retorted.

I flushed.

"I'm doing what I was trained to do and what the law demands of me," I said. "I cannot just refill your medicines blindly."

"You're a quack! You're worthless! Why would a doctor end up in Hotspur? We get those that can't make it anywhere else! You even got kicked out of the hospital so you have to make house calls!"

"I was reinstated yesterday. I did nothing wrong, but another doctor doubted me. I was right, he was wrong. Now I don't have to do home visits," I said, controlling my anger.

"Then why are you here?" she asked.

"Because Tommy and Agatha Templar asked me to come

and see you," I replied. "I'm here to help you. Do you want my help or should I leave?"

Sarah looked at Willis.

"You're out of medicine and it will be days before Dr. Tarnasky can see you in Dallas," Willis pleaded.

Sarah looked unhappy.

"Please, darling!" Willis implored.

Sarah nodded.

"Go ahead, Doc!" Willis said.

I opened my briefcase and took out my stethoscope and blood pressure machine and laid them on the table. I read the labels on her bottles.

"You're on glyburide for diabetes, and lisinopril for high blood pressure and to protect your kidneys from diabetes," I said. "And you take pravastatin to control your cholesterol. Why do you take valproic acid?"

She looked away.

"Do you have seizures or depression?" I asked.

"You're the doctor, you figure it out," she said.

"She has depression, Doc," Mr. Woodcox said.

"I read your reports from Dallas. You're in pretty good health, it seems. No major surgeries other than a hysterectomy. No allergies, no family history, no other medical problems. Is that right?"

She shook her head.

"May I examine you?" I asked.

"Do I need to undress?" she asked, alarmed.

"No."

I checked her blood pressure; it was normal. I smelled cigarette smoke on her breath. The skin of her arms was thin and wrinkled. She had a thick patina of make-up, especially around her eyes. She had a small ear ring on the inner rim of her right ear. Her teeth were stained brown and her gums were swollen. I listened to her heart and lungs and palpated her abdomen. Her heart rate was irregular and I heard wheezing in her lungs. I checked her knee and biceps reflexes, and tested for sensation; they were intact.

I straightened up.

"You must have been taking Dilantin or phenytoin or a Anjalilar agent for depression for at least six months," I said.

"How do you know that?" Sarah asked.

"Your gums are swollen. That's seen with Dilantin after you take it for several months."

She nodded and kept staring at me.

"Have you found anything else?" she asked.

"You smoke and have emphysema."

She laughed hoarsely.

"You don't have to be a genius to figure *that* out," she said.

"You used to suffer from right sided migraines, but now they're better."

She was surprised.

"And how do you know that?" she asked.

"You have that little earring on the right. Many people have that done for migraines. It must have worked because you're not on any particular treatment for migraines now."

She covered her right ear protectively and glared.

"I would like to check your radial pulse, at the wrist. Please remove your right glove," I requested.

She jerked back.

"No!" she cried.

Willis came up to me.

"Why? Why is that necessary?" he asked, concerned.

"Mrs. Woodcox has an irregular pulse," I explained. "This could be due to atrial fibrillation, but it is not as irregular as I expect with fibrillation. She may have emphysema of the lungs, and the air trapping can cause some pulsations to get suppressed. So I need to check the radial pulse at the wrist to see what's going on."

They looked at each other.

"No one has ever said that before," she said and looked away.

"Please remove your glove so I can check your pulse," I repeated. "It won't take long."

"Absolutely not!" she said angrily and crossed her hands on her lap.

There was an awkward pause.

"It's not painful," I said. "Just takes a minute to check your pulse."

"No! I said no! I let you do the exam! Now fill my medicines and leave!"

Mr. Woodcox stepped in.

"Sarah, darling," he said, softly, "maybe you should let him."

"No!"

"Then he can be done."

"No!"

"Darling, he's a doctor. Let him finish."

"No!"

Mr. Woodcox turned to me.

"Would you give us a moment? I need to talk to her. Leave your things here," he said.

I walked to the front door. The atrium was lined with the same yellow crepe wallpaper. I noticed a heap of rolled up newspapers in the corner and unopened mail stacked up on a side table. The wood flooring was muddy and scratched. I noticed my jacket and felt for my cell phone.

"You need to make a call?" Mr. Woodcox asked, reappearing.
I turned.

"I was going to call my wife and tell her I'll be late."

"Cell phones are high. Don't waste your money. Use our land line later. Penny saved is a penny earned."

He nodded towards the living room.

"She's agreed to let you check her pulse," he said.

I walked back.

Mrs. Woodcox looked away. As I approached she slowly pulled her gloves off.

There were several slash marks on her wrists, more on the left than the right. Some were thin and superficial, but a few on the left were thick, jagged, and had required stitches. There was a neat scar of a surgical repair of the left radial artery.

I said nothing.

"Say it, doctor!" she cried. "You can say it!"

"What do you mean?" I asked.

"Say it! Say, I see you slashed your wrists! Say, I see you tried to kill yourself! Say it!"

"What happened in the past is none of my business. I'm going to check your pulses," I said. "Please take a deep breath and hold it."

I checked the pulses at the wrists. The left pulse was weak and thready but the right one was strong. The pulses diminished when she took a deep breath and held it in.

"You do have emphysema, probably from smoking," I said. "Air is getting trapped in your lungs and suppresses some of your heart beats."

She nodded, and wiped her eyes.

"You really should stop smoking," I said.

She shook her head.

"Even though you have lung damage, you could limit it by

quitting."

Sarah looked away.

"It can cause lung cancer," I added.

"You know what I say to cancer? *Bring it on!* I don't care if I get cancer! Every day is a living hell!"

I was taken aback.

"I wish I were already dead! I couldn't even kill myself! Willis is always on edge that he might let me out of his sight for a minute and I'll go kill myself! Isn't that right, darling?"

Willis was quiet.

"Oh, you can say it, darling. You've hidden all the handguns. The big kitchen knives are all gone. I know you're watching me," Sarah said.

"I love you and I know you are an intelligent woman," he said.

There was a silence.

"Everyone wants to hear it. Everyone wants to know, what's that rich little girl from Dallas gone and done now? They're *so* curious. Why did she want to kill herself? How did she try to do it? Who stitched her up and saved her? The Gillettes and the Novicheks and the Marshalls would love to hear all the details, wouldn't they?"

Willis hugged her neck.

"You're not in Dallas, darling. No one there knows anything. Don't worry."

Willis turned to me.

"Sarah grew up in Fort Worth but her family moved to Dallas. Very famous, well known family. Sarah wants this issue to remain private."

I nodded. We heard the wind rattle the windows and spray them with dirt.

"That be the haboob," Willis noted. "Terrible thing

happened in Jarrell, terrible. Bad timing, having the Chamber lunch today."

Sarah defiantly took out a pack of cigarettes.

"I will write out all your medicines. I can read the doses from the bottles."

"Thank you, Doc," Willis said.

I wrote out the prescriptions and handed them over. I packed my briefcase and stood up.

"Goodbye, Dr. Mathur," Mrs. Woodcox said, coldly. "See you at the Chamber lunch."

"I'll walk you out," Mr. Woodcox said.

I picked up my jacket and we walked down to the gate. The air was thicker and I tasted sand as I spoke.

"Supposed to have a big dust storm blow in from Lubbock today," I repeated, not knowing what to say. I straightened a birdbath. It was marbled with soil and bird droppings.

"Yard's a mess," Willis said.

"Looks like you haven't had much time for it," I said.

"Been taking Sarah to Dallas a bunch."

"Last year's winter flowers are still in the beds, and the lantana has all but died off. You started to put some rye grass in but didn't finish. Looks like she got really sick last winter," I guessed.

Mr. Woodcox stopped and stared at me.

"Who told you? Tommy?" he demanded.

"What do you mean? Tommy didn't tell me anything," I exclaimed. "It just looks like you haven't had time for your yard since last winter. I'm guessing your wife's had depression since then, for which you've been taking her to Dallas."

Mr. Woodcox opened the gate. He swallowed and looked away.

"You're right," he said.

"Depression is nothing to be ashamed of. There is a lot of depression in my own family," I said. "It's a disease, due to loss of some particular chemicals in the brain."

Willis said nothing.

"I tell everyone, depression is common and it's nothing to be ashamed about. It's a chemical deficiency disease, like diabetes, and needs treatment."

Willis hesitated, then spoke.

"She was not a depressive person, Doc, she doesn't have regular depression," he said quietly.

He opened the gate and paused on the sidewalk. I walked to my car.

"I'll see you at the Chamber lunch," I said, trying to change the subject. I got in.

Mr. Woodcox tapped the passenger side window. I leaned over and rolled it down.

"I guess you'll find out anyhow," he said. "She doesn't have regular depression, Doc. She's not depressed on account of lack of chemicals in the brain. She's depressed on account of our son killed himself last Christmas."

He turned and walked away briskly through the swirling dust.

CHAPTER 10

THE KNIFE OF THE PARTY

The Hotspur Chamber of Commerce is located on the corner of Commercial Avenue and Pecan, across from Falcon Pharmacy. It is an elongated rectangular corner building with an all-glass front and a side wall decorated with all the brands of the cattle ranches of the county. I was late; there was no parking spot on either street. I parked near the drugstore and hurried out. The wind whistled around me; sharp grains of dust scratched my eyes and face as I scrambled up the sidewalk. The Chamber was packed; as I entered, I heard a familiar voice over the clamor.

"I'm so glad you made it!" Andrea Godwyn greeted me.

"Yes. Fortunately, your husband did not call me back to the ER, so here I am," I said.

Andrea held up a hand in warning.

"Simon said he's busy, so he may be fixing to call you. Better get something to eat. We've got finger sandwiches and little sausages and pecan chocolates. All the food's local, of course."

"Thanks, I'm really hungry."

"Maya is over here," she said, and I followed her. Maya was wearing a striking crimson dress and garnet earrings. She was talking to a tall, slender lady in a bright green pantsuit and large sunglasses. I noticed she had a large hearing aid with a wire leading to a device in a shirt pocket.

"This is my husband, Sandip," Maya said, "and this is Jane Pettenguard. She's a reporter from Dallas."

We shook hands. Jane Pettenguard had long white hair which she stroked over her hearing aid. She pursed her lips and stared at me expectantly. I spoke up hastily.

"All the way from Dallas? That's a rather long drive," I said.

"This Chamber sends us a nice invitation every year, so the editor said, all right, all right, let's go check it out," she said, drawing out her words. "Poor me. I was the unlucky one. Had to come driving down here in this God-awful dust storm to this God-forsaken hellhole in God-knows-where."

Maya and I exchanged glances.

"I get the feeling you're not thrilled to be here," I ventured.

She lifted up her glasses and rubbed her left eye vigorously. I saw that it was red.

"I've got something in my eye; don't worry, Jane, it's nothing," she said.

"Have you been driving around the county?" I asked.

"Yes," she answered. "Not much to write about. But you're the English doctor I've heard about."

"Actually, I'm not English. I'm from India. I did train in London for four years, though."

"You have a British accent," she said.

"We are all shocked by the news about Princess Diana," Jane said. "She just died in a car wreck, you know."

"We heard," Maya said. "I understand she was trying to avoid the press."

Jane stared at her.

"Yes, they hounded her and made her life miserable," I added.

"We're not all like that," Jane declared.

I shrugged. She lifted her glasses and rubbed her eye again.

"It'll go away in time, I'm sure," she said.

Her tone changed to a silky whisper.

"Oh, aren't you the one who set a poor patient on fire?" she asked, pleasantly.

I was taken aback. Ms. Pettenguard blinked, feigning

surprise.

"Oh, I shouldn't have said that. Maybe that's a sore point — silly, silly Jane," she said, still watching me intently.

I was shocked. I glanced at Maya. She was scowling.

"I *never* set anyone on fire! What happened was an accident by another doctor, not me. The hospital board and the State Board had a joint inquiry, and they cleared me," I said, angrily.

Jane Pettenguard grasped my arm and made a face of elaborate contrition.

"I'm *so* sorry, I didn't mean to offend you. It was my understanding that *you* were the one who, you know, set a patient on fire," she went on sweetly. "Heavens above! Setting a patient on fire! Any comments, Doctor?"

"I can't discuss it. Patient confidentiality," I said firmly.

"Do you have anything to say?" she asked. "Anything at all?"

She dropped her voice dramatically.

"Off the record?" she whispered.

I shook my head.

"I really didn't mean to offend you," she repeated, smiling. "Silly, silly Jane."

"Please excuse us," I said, and Maya and I turned away and went back to the buffet. We ate in silence for a few minutes.

"What a nasty woman!" I burst out. Maya looked over my shoulder.

"She's heading towards the Woodcoxes," Maya said. "Didn't you just see them for a home visit?"

"Yes, Mrs. Woodcox wanted some medicines refilled. I thought we were going to see the Rutherfords here," I said.

"So did I," Maya nodded. "You know, Patty Rutherford came to our house that night because she found another jacket that she thought I would like. You had gone back to the hospital."

"She drove down from her ranch? At night?"

"Yes. It was ten o'clock. She was full of energy! She wouldn't come in, just handed me the jacket and shot off."

"She keeps her ranch humming. I don't think her husband does much," I said.

"True. I called the next day to thank her and he said she had gone to California. He was watching television at ten in the morning."

"So he doesn't worry about the ranch too much," I said.

"Agatha just waved to me. Let's go meet the Templars," Maya suggested. We wove our way through the crowd, holding our plates and glasses aloft.

"Did you ask them about the Rutherfords?" I asked.

"Agatha told me they had a son, but she didn't want to talk about it, so don't ask," Maya whispered.

We met the Templars and they introduced us to their friends and business partners.

"Sandi is the new doctor here," Tommy said, thumping me on the back. "And he's a good one! I've stopped going to Scott and White. I'm going to stay with him!"

"I second that," Agatha chirped. "Sandi and Maya are a real asset to our little community."

A tall man with thick blond hair offered his hand.

"Travis Parrish, from Waxahachie, pleased to meet you. Believe you know my parents, Roger and Gwen," he smiled.

"Yes, I do! Your parents were my hosts for Thanksgiving. Maya and our daughters were in Canada."

"You had a good time with them?"

"Pretty good. I made a small mistake, but I think they forgave me," I said.

"You're the one who brought a bottle of wine? For a Church Of Christ preacher?" Travis asked, grinning.

"Guilty," I admitted.

"Bet you never even heard of the Church of Christ and such in London, Doc! It's okay, no way you could have known. They got a real kick out of it. Bonnie wondered what the neighbors thought, seeing you bring a giant bottle of wine to a Church of Christ preacher!" Travis laughed. The Templars shook their heads, amused.

Andrea appeared again.

"Simon called. He needs you in the ER. They just brought in someone who's semiconscious," she said.

"I'll be right there," I sighed. I put down my plate and ice tea and hugged Maya quickly. As I headed out, I walked past Jane Pettenguard. She had cornered the Woodcoxes and they looked very uncomfortable. The area around the three of them was curiously vacant, and there was palpable tension as Jane Pettenguard spoke in a stage whisper. She edged closer to Mr. Woodcox.

"I'm curious. So *why* did you resign as mayor? You had just six months left. Why not finish it out?" she asked, skewering fruit with a toothpick.

"I had some personal reasons," Mr. Woodcox said.

"Something you wish to share? Something the public ought to know?" Jane persisted. "Or just tell me off the record? Totally confidential, of course."

"How was your drive down from Dallas, darling?" Mrs. Woodcox asked, her voice sharp. "I know you met our state trooper. Speeding? Couldn't wait to get here?"

Jane spun around and studied Mrs. Woodcox.

"Were *you* the personal reason, darling?" she asked. "Poor me, I don't know anything, I'm such an outsider, I just have to ask!"

The Woodcoxes looked around, anticipating escape.

Jane took off her glasses and rubbed her eye vigorously.

"Oh, that really burns!" she mumbled.

I seized my chance.

"Mrs. Pettenguard, you may have a serious issue with your eye," I said. "Come with me, I'm going to the ER. I'll take a look at your eye."

Jane Pettenguard shook her head.

"It's not that bad. I'm talking to Willis and Sarah Louise Woodcox, and I have so much to catch up with them. So many of my readers in Dallas would like to know about them," she turned to them and beamed. They looked disgusted.

"Sarah Louise is from old oil money, you know, so I said, Jane, Jane, you have to tell her story," Jane fretted and squinted at Sarah. She suddenly grabbed Sarah's wrist and Sarah gasped. I stepped in between them and Sarah jerked free.

"Miss Pettenguard, I'm serious. You could have a piece of grit in your cornea. I can take a look and see if you've damaged your cornea," I insisted.

"No thank you."

"It could affect your vision permanently," I warned.

"Seriously?"

"It could cause blindness," I insisted.

"I don't believe you," she said flatly.

"Suit yourself. I'm going to the ER, I already have a patient there. Don't wait too long. Remember, you could damage your eye permanently!" I turned towards the door.

Jane wavered.

"Don't go blind," I called out.

"Wait!" she called.

I turned.

"Are you serious? I could have permanent eye damage?" she asked again.

"You've been rubbing your eye repeatedly, and your eye is

pretty inflamed. Go to the bathroom, see for yourself," I said.

"But I'm not done with these precious people!" she wailed, theatrically.

Mr. and Mrs. Woodcox took a few steps back.

"Your eye is very inflamed, you could lose vision," I repeated, sternly.

Jane Pettenguard wavered, then decided.

"Oh, all right! It really is burning a lot!" she admitted.

She turned to the Woodcoxes. They had begun to walk away with great haste.

"*Well!*" she pouted. She put down her plate and grabbed her purse and followed me hastily to the door.

I looked back.

Mrs. Woodcox turned at that moment and mouthed *thank you*. Jane followed me out the door.

"I really wanted to meet the Rutherfords. I knew their son," she said.

"You did?" I said.

"Yes. He was a friend of a friend, in college," she said.

"Where is he now?"

"Don't know, last I heard, San Francisco. I know where your hospital is, Dr. Mathur. Go ahead, I'll see you there."

I shuffled into the ER.

"Dr. Mathur! So sorry to pull you away from the Chamber lunch!" Simon said, "but we've got this fellow here and he's unresponsive!"

The ER reeked of stale clothes and urine. There were two gurneys in the room, and a tall, gaunt man was stretched out on one of them. He had matted hair, a full beard, and skin layered and fissured with hardened sweat and dirt. He wore overalls stiff with oil stains and no shirt. He breathed irregularly through an open mouth with four teeth. I glanced at the monitor.

"So he's got a blood pressure of eighty by sixty, and a pulse of a hundred and six, and at least he's breathing," I observed. "So what's the story?"

"He was discovered by his pastor, Mr. Roger Parrish, whom I believe you are acquainted with," Simon smiled. "The offering of the colossal wine bottle to the fiercely abstinent?"

"Yes, I just met their son, who also reminded me, thank you," I said, drily. "Simon, why are there two gurneys in this room?"

"Oh, the roof in Exam Room Two collapsed last night. Luckily, no one was there. So we cleaned the gurney and moved it here, in case we had two patients," Simon explained.

"The last time we closed Room Two, it was because there was a power failure due to squirrels nibbling the wires," I recalled.

"Truth is stranger than fiction, is it not?"

"Yes. You can't make this stuff up."

"I hear you have another patient coming in," Simon said.

"Yes, and unfortunately she's a nosy reporter from Dallas. She's trying to dig up dirt on everyone. Now she has to be in this room with the other patient!"

"You anticipate she will be distressed at the prospect of sharing a room with a comatose, malodorous gent?"

"Yes, I do. Well, at least she wasn't in Exam Room Two when the roof fell in," I said.

Simon shrugged

"Pity," he smiled wryly.

I nodded.

"Do we have any information on this man here?" I asked. Simon handed me a clipboard.

"The Right Honorable Ulysses Best, Esquire," he announced.

"Ulysses Best," I summarized. "Forty-two, single, works for Wilson Pipeline Services, no medicines, no allergies, no surgeries. History of heavy alcohol abuse. Mr. Parrish kept checking on him and thought that Ulysses had stopped drinking. Somehow, our patient found a way to obtain his nectar. Mr. Parrish found him unconscious in his trailer and called the ambulance. What's this about a cat?"

"Oh, there was a rather miserable mangy cat there, too, in the gentleman's trailer. The paramedics took pity on it and brought it in. Raggedy little bugger, shivering and scared out of its senses. I wrapped it in a towel and gave it some milk and set it down outside by the Coke machine."

I unbuttoned the man's overalls and examined him. There was a sudden stench of urine and rotten food, and a faint sweet smell in his breath.

"His neck and face are covered over with dirt and oil, guess he doesn't wash too often," I observed. "Watch out for lice and bedbugs. His heart and lungs are clear, but he's breathing pretty irregularly. He doesn't smell of alcohol, that's surprising. His breath actually smells *sweet*. That's odd."

"True, I didn't smell alcohol either," Simon said.

"Call the paramedics and ask them if they found any vodka bottles. Vodka doesn't make your breath smell. All the alcoholics like it for that reason. Also ask Mr. Parrish if there were any liquor bottles in the trash. Tell him to go back to the trailer and check."

"Do you really need to know all that?" Simon asked.

"I may need to transfer him," I explained. "I want to be sure about the facts. Ask Mr. Parrish to check the trash cans of the neighboring trailers as well, because many alcoholics throw their bottles in other peoples' trash cans."

There was a knock on the door. Jane Pettenguard stood

there with an admission form in one hand and covered her bad eye with the other.

"Come in, Mrs. Pettenguard," I said. "This is Simon Godwyn, RN, the ER nurse. He will check you in."

"Surely I am going to the other room?" she asked.

"Unfortunately, that room is not operational," Simon announced. "Consequently, I shall endeavor to care for you here, madam."

Jane Pettenguard peered at Simon with dislike.

"Oh, another English accent! Hotspur's got a very English hospital!" she sneered.

"A shrewd observation, madam! I will take your admission form. Would you kindly sit here on the side of the gurney, facing away from the gentleman? I shall check your vital signs and prepare your encounter form."

"I hope you're not going to undress me," Jane said, mischievously.

Simon flushed.

"Not at all, madam," he stammered.

"Or undress the gentleman," she went on, "though it won't bother me, really."

"I believe you have an issue with your left eye, madam," Simon responded. "I don't believe that requires you to disrobe."

"Well, let me know if you just *want* me to disrobe," she added slyly, to Simon's discomfiture.

She smiled. She was enjoying making Simon squirm.

I returned to my examination. Ulysses moaned a little but did not protest as I palpated his abdomen. It was sunken, but the liver was enlarged. I checked the area around the neck and found several red spots. The man's limbs were flaccid and he did not respond to commands.

"Did you see all the red spots around his neck, Simon?" I

asked.

"Yes," he answered, "I wondered about that."

"Those are signs of liver damage," I explained. "But they look old. I'm still worried that there's no smell of alcohol. Let's check the blood and ask for an alcohol level and a urinary drug screen."

"Will be with you in a jiffy!" Simon answered, as he finished preparing Jane Pettenguard.

"And don't forget to call the paramedics and Roger Parrish."

Simon and a paramedic, David, dragged a flimsy screen between the two patients. They peeled the overalls off Ulysses and gaped at his underwear. His shorts were crisp with waste; they were cut open and gingerly extracted, sealed in a plastic bag, and carried out. Ulysses was gaunt, his translucent skin draped his skull and skeleton like cling film. His wasted muscles were as thin as the tendons that connected them to his warped joints. He breathed irregularly, sometimes deeply and sometimes, barely at all. I smelled his breath again; still, the strange sweet odor but no smell of alcohol.

"Ask Tom to rush his labs and get a urinalysis and urine drug screen," I ordered.

"I've sent the blood test but there wasn't any urine."

"Then you'll have to catheterize him."

Simon groaned.

"He's filthy, Doctor! Have you seen his skin?"

"I'm sorry, Simon. We need a urine sample."

Simon grunted. He took Jane Pettenguard's clipboard and handed it to me.

"She's ready for you," he said.

"I'll get started with her while you get ready for the catheterization."

"Marvelous," Simon said, scowling. "Splendid."

I stopped thinking about Ulysses and glanced at the clipboard.

"Mrs. Janice Ogilvy Pettenguard, of Highland Park, Dallas, fifty-seven years old," I read aloud. Jane winced.

"Do you really have to *announce* that?" she snapped.

"You're on captopril and hydrochlorothiazide twice daily for hypertension, and you take a baby aspirin daily," I read out. "Hysterectomy, gall bladder surgery and appendectomy. Negative heart catheterization, that's good. Allergic to codeine and hydrocodone. You smoke half a pack a day and drink socially. Correct so far?"

"That's me," she agreed.

"Let me examine you. Just stay sitting up," I said.

I examined her briskly. Everything was normal except for the inflamed eye.

"Do you want to see the scars on my belly?" she asked.

"No, you're not having any abdominal problems, and you're not tender there."

"I'm not shy," she reiterated, "even though I'm with two foreign men."

"Just lie down and let me put in some eye drops. The drops will numb the lining. Then I'm going to stain your eye with fluorescein," I explained.

"What's that?" she asked.

"It's a yellow stain that makes the whole eye turn yellow but any scratches turn bright green. That way I can see if there's a scratch on the clear part of the eye, the cornea, and see if there's a foreign body stuck at the end of that scratch."

"Will it hurt?"

"It might sting a little as the numbing drops go in," I said, and helped her lie flat. I draped a towel over her neck and upper chest.

"That's so the dye doesn't get onto your nice dress," I explained.

"Oscar de la Renta," she said.

"Very nice. I'm going to pull your lower eyelid down and first irrigate your eye with saline, just to moisten it all up. You will feel the saline running down the side of your face," I warned her.

"Wait! Let me take my hearing aid off," she said. "Don't want water in it."

She removed it and handed both parts to me. They were larger and heavier than I expected. I placed them in a plastic bag and dropped the bag into her purse.

"It's in your purse," I informed her.

I adjusted the overhead lights and slipped on sterile gloves. I pulled down the lower eyelid.

"Look up, towards your forehead," I instructed, and squirted saline.

"Whoa!" she shuddered, but remained lying down.

"Now I'm going to put in the drops."

"Go for it!"

I dripped in the lidocaine drops carefully, avoiding overflow.

"Now close your eyes, let the medicine work," I said.

Simon cleared his throat.

"Dr. Mathur, I need to catheterize Mr. Ulysses," he said, uncomfortably. "Would you please come back here to supervise?"

I looked at him through the feeble fabric.

"Don't we have a better screen? This one is almost transparent," I complained.

"This is all we have. But I could hang a couple of bedsheets over it," he offered.

"Don't worry about me," Jane declared. "I'm not looking. Mind you, it won't bother me, seeing a naked man."

"Do you think you could put *several* sheets over the frame?" I asked Simon, sharply.

"I've been to a nude beach in France," Jane continued happily, "and I've seen everything, Doctor. I mean, *everything!*"

She relished the uncomfortable silence.

"You two are such prudes! So British! You know why you don't see naked men all over the place?" she asked, her voice vibrant.

"No," I said, trying to sound disinterested.

"Naked men don't look good. They're *irregular*. Lumpy. Asymmetrical. Women, on the other hand, are smooth and symmetrical," she explained, triumphantly. "They look good naked."

"A succinct summary of anatomy," Simon declared.

"I think men look good in briefs, but look terrible when they take them off. Never went back to the nudist beach, never," Jane said. "Too traumatic."

Simon and I moved to Ulysses. Simon gently pulled the hospital gown back. His groin was matted with dirt and feces. Simon held his breath and cleaned him, then placed towels all around. He opened a catheterization set, put on a gown, pulled on sterile gloves, and grasped the Foley catheter. I supervised the exercise.

"What size Foley?" I asked.

"I'm using a twenty-two French," Simon answered.

"Hah! I knew it," Jane declared. "The French have everything to do with sex."

"It's just the diameter of the catheter, madam," Simon said. "It has nothing to do with sex."

"Oh, I've hurt your British feelings, have I? I'm so sorry, my dear chap! But you're in Texas now, dear fellow, and all your royal manners have to go! They must go! Texas is a no-bullshit state,

Lord Simon!" Jane went on, her voice shrill.

Simon shook his head. He inserted the catheter deeply.

"I'm in the bladder, but there's no urine. He's dry," he said.

"Increase the IV fluids. Give him five hundred cc now, wide open. Inflate the balloon and leave the Foley in place so we can catch any urine he makes. Call the paramedics and Roger Parrish again," I ordered. "We've got to find out what's happening with this man!"

Simon disappeared into the dictation room and started calling.

Jane Pettenguard had her eyes closed, and was smiling blissfully.

"How much longer do I have to wait? This room smells like an animal stall!" she said.

"Another few minutes," I answered.

"So you trained in London?" she asked.

"Yes."

"Then in Houston?"

"Yes."

"How do you like it here, far away from all the big hospitals?"

"It's very different."

"Bet you can't wait to get back," she needled.

"Well, it's been interesting. I've had to rely on the basics. Look for clues, manage with limited labs," I explained.

Simon stepped out, phone in hand.

"Phone's not working," he said.

"There's a loose wire in the jack."

"Got it. Brilliant," Simon muttered.

Jane smiled condescendingly as Simon struggled, then got through. He reappeared.

"Tom says they can't do the alcohol level. The machine's broken," he announced.

I moved up to him.

"Okay, do the chemistry panel, and save the sample," I hissed. "Any news from the paramedics or Sam?"

"No, but I'm still trying."

Jane cleared her throat. She had heard everything.

"I see what you mean. You have to go with your gut, your best guess," Jane continued. "Your lab is pretty useless. Can't even do a simple alcohol level."

I flushed.

"It's not useless. They do the best they can. A doctor has to look for clues, and ask questions," I said, and returned to her side. I was irritated.

"You think you're a medical Sherlock Holmes, right?" she said, and snorted.

"You know, Sherlock Holmes *was* based on a professor of medicine."

"Really? I knew that Conan Doyle was a doctor," Jane said.

"The character of Sherlock Holmes was based on Sir Conan Doyle's professor of medicine in Edinburgh, Dr. Bell," I said.

"So what have you deduced about me?" Jane asked, blinking her eyes and looking at me.

"Let me put in the fluorescein," I countered.

I opened a sealed packet and took out a thin strip of paper. It had a yellow bead.

"I want you to look up towards your forehead again," I instructed.

I rolled down her lower eyelid and touched it with the yellow tip. The stain spread rapidly into the moisture.

"Now close your eyes and move them around from side to side," I said.

I grasped a pair of magnifying glasses and plugged in an ultraviolet lamp. It beamed blue light.

"Now I'm going to examine your cornea. Look straight up at the ceiling and hold still," I said.

The cornea was an even blue, but there was a bright green streak at the one o'clock position. I looked carefully at the track.

"You've got an abrasion, and I think there's a foreign body there at the end of the scratch. It must have hit at an angle, like a meteor, and it's embedded at the deep end of the scratch," I said.

"Like a meteor," Jane repeated. "I like your comparisons."

I pulsed the abrasion with a jet of sterile water, trying to flush the particle out.

"No luck," I said. "I'm going to use the tip of a needle. Hold very still!"

"Is this safe?" Jane asked. "Should you be doing this? Poking my eye with a needle? Here, in Hotspur?"

"I'm going to try to dislodge it with the tip of a twenty-five gauge needle. If that piece stays there, your eye will not heal and the cornea may perforate before you can get to Dallas," I said, pulling back.

"What do you mean, perforate?" she asked, alarmed.

"You could develop a hole in the front of your eye. Then the water in your eye would leak out of your eye and the inside of your eye could get infected," I explained.

She shuddered.

"Go ahead. Be careful," she said.

I peered at the deep end of the abrasion. I took the sharp end of the needle and inserted it gently. I flicked the tip and felt it scratch something hard.

"I can feel the surface of the particle," I said. "There's definitely something stuck there. I'm going to try again."

This time I went fractionally deeper and at a glancing angle. The tip of the needle jammed into something hard. I pushed a little.

Nothing.

My mouth dried up and I felt my heart pound.

I pushed again, at a different angle.

Nothing.

I pushed again, and twisted the needle like a screwdriver.

The membrane heaved, and suddenly the tip of the fragment stuck out of the groove. I nudged the end and slowly teased it out. It wobbled onto the side of the gorge it had created.

"Quickly! Give me five cc of sterile water!" I cried. "Now!"

Simon snapped open a vial and drew it up. I grabbed it and flushed the metal away until it lay just outside the cornea, the transparent part of the eye.

"Magnet!" I called out. "Give me a magnet!"

"We don't have a magnet, doctor!" Simon replied.

"Give me the large round magnet we use to disable pacemakers. It's on the crash cart."

Simon found it and handed it to me.

"It's not sterile," he noted.

"I'm not going to touch the eye," I reassured him, "just hold it above the metal."

I held the magnet just above the fragment.

Nothing.

"It's some other metal, not iron. Give me a piece of cotton!"

I changed gloves and pulled a piece of cotton wool into a strand, and made it into a U. I twisted the bottom of the U over the fragment, and lifted it up gingerly.

The fragment came off perfectly.

"I think I got it out!" I whooped.

"You *think?*" Jane asked, stiffly.

"I'm pretty sure. Let me flush and take another look."

I irrigated the eye with saline and looked again. The fullness at the deep end was gone. I watched the wound carefully, not daring to breathe. No internal fluid welled up.

"I think we're good! No sign of a perforation!" I declared.

Jane sighed with relief.

"Now what?" she asked.

"Just relax, I'm going to flush your eye and put some antibiotic ointment, then close your eye for a couple of days to let the cornea heal. You can see your local doctor to make sure it's healing, but it looks good," I said.

I squeezed Neosporin ointment into her eye and made her close her eyes and then move her eyeballs around, to spread the Neosporin. I placed a gauze pad over her left eye and taped it in place. I sat her up cautiously.

"You can open your other eye," I said.

She blinked.

"It feels better," she admitted.

"Good, I'm glad. Let's get you out of here. I need to concentrate on my other patient," I said.

"Actually, I want to stay and see what happens to the other patient," Jane announced.

"You can't do that!" I protested.

"Sure I can, it's a public interest story," Jane said.

"It's just a patient in a small hospital," I said. "He's entitled to his privacy."

"Not just any little hospital in Texas," Jane said evenly. "The *British* Hospital of Texas. I want to see what we can expect from you foreigners."

CHAPTER 11

THE GREAT BRITISH HOSPITAL OF TEXAS

"That's unfair," I said, angrily. "You have no business hanging around now. We've taken care of you, we're done! You should leave immediately. Go back to Dallas."

"This hospital is falling apart. It should be closed! It's beyond repair," Jane declared.

"We took care of you! Everything worked out!" I protested.

"Just lucky. You can't keep muddling on. This hospital should be closed!" Jane said.

"The people need the hospital," I argued, restraining myself. "We just started making money again."

"Why hadn't it made money before?" she asked.

I hesitated.

"They couldn't bill insurance because the doctor who did all the admissions never wrote a single discharge summary for three years!"

"That's ridiculous! How could the hospital survive three years without billing insurance?"

"Bank loans, donations, unpaid debts. They didn't pay their staff for three months," I said.

"You have no real lab, no CT scanner, no ultrasound, and a bare bones ER with one room!" Jane snapped. "This hospital should be closed!"

"We make it work!" I snapped back.

"With what?"

"With whatever we have!"

"You have nothing! I mean, you have no computers here.

What do you know about me? How are you going to send my information to my doctor?"

"We'll get electronic records eventually. We have other priorities. We will send your records by fax," I answered.

"You know nothing about me," she repeated. "And you operated on me!"

"It was a minor procedure, not an operation. And I do know a fair amount about you," I countered.

"What do you know about me?" Jane asked and stood up, holding on to the edge of the gurney. She glared at me with her good eye.

"There's nothing wrong with your hearing," I said. "You took off your hearing aid and you heard me whisper to Simon. I bet that's a recording device."

Jane was silent for a minute.

"Go on," she said, quietly.

"You have money problems. You live in Highland Park, but you have a Bronze health plan with insurance I've never heard of, and you take old medicines. You're wearing de la Renta, but there are food stains on it, you didn't get it professionally cleaned. Your shoes are worn and repaired. Oh, your car inspection sticker expired three months ago," I said. "Looks like trouble in paradise."

Jane was shocked.

"How dare you! You're incredibly rude and obnoxious, Doctor!" she cried. "Just for that, I will sit outside and see what happens to this patient. God help you if you can't help him!"

She grabbed her purse and stormed outside.

Simon reappeared from the dictation room and grinned.

"She deserved it," he said.

We looked at Ulysses. He was still unresponsive.

"Roger found one bottle of vodka in his trash," Simon said.

"That's not a lot," I said. "Doesn't account for this level of sedation."

I looked at his labs.

"Can Tom send the sample to Brownwood?" I asked.

"No carrier."

"Let's do some detective work. Look at the blood chemistry. See, the positive ions, sodium and potassium should be almost equal to the negative ones, chloride and bicarbonate. The normal difference is around fourteen. What are his chemistries?"

"Sodium plus potassium is one-fifty-four and chloride plus bicarb is one-twenty," Simon calculated.

"So there is a gap of thirty-four," I said. "There's got to be some chemical causing that big gap. Could be alcohol, but there's no smell. Could be body acids retained due to kidney failure, but his kidney numbers are just barely elevated."

"That slight elevation of the kidney tests could be due to dehydration," Simon said.

"True, but you had already given him almost a liter of fluids before they drew the blood. There's got to be some chemical, some poison, that's causing that big gap in his blood chemistry. I'm worried about anti-freeze," I said.

"Anti-freeze?" Simon asked, surprised.

"Roger had been riding him about alcohol. Maybe he drank what vodka he could get, then got some anti-freeze. Many alcoholics do that. Makes the breath smell sweet," I said.

"So what would we do differently?" Simon asked. "We just need to watch him, rehydrate him and keep his airway clear?"

"No, we might need to send him for dialysis. The anti-freeze can plug up his kidneys and put him into severe renal failure," I explained.

"So his kidneys will shut down?"

"Yes. Maybe that's why he isn't making any urine."

"Well, good luck trying to transfer him! We're in a real pickle here. The big hospitals in Dallas won't be willing to take an uninsured patient."

"Especially without any conclusive lab data to prove it," I agreed.

"How can we prove that he took anti-freeze? They will want proof, some proof, before they take him. Pretty bloody hopeless!" Simon shook his head.

I imagined Jane Pettenguard outside, thirsting for revenge.

"Call St. Paul's in Fort Worth. They take a lot of charity cases for their medical students. Let me check his eyes to see if there's any damage. Methyl alcohol can do all of this, too."

I examined the eyes with a fundoscope, to check the inner lining of the eye.

"Anything wrong with the retina?" Simon asked.

"Nothing," I admitted.

"I was hoping you would find something, something to justify the transfer," Simon said.

"Me, too," I agreed. "Any urine in the bag?"

Simon checked.

"Nothing," he declared.

"Another bad sign, he's still not making urine. There's definitely something wrong here! I bet he's been drinking anti-freeze, I'm sure that's the problem, but we need something to back us up!" I was desperate.

There was a knock at the door. It was Jane, with a limp grey kitten swaddled in a towel.

"There's a cat that's starving," she said. "I found it by the Coke machine. Can I get some food or milk for it?"

"It came with this patient," Simon rushed forward and took the limp bundle.

"The towel is reeking with cat pee!" Jane sneered. "Perhaps

you could find her a dry towel? *If* your hospital can spare it?"

We ignored her and Simon peeled the wet towel off the cat. We sat her down on a fresh towel in the corner and Simon threw the wet one in the trash.

"Hold on!" I said. "I just thought of something!"

I turned to make sure that Jane had left.

"Give me the Wood's light!" I said.

"You mean, the one you just used for Mrs. Pattenguard?" Simon asked, puzzled.

"Yes! And turn the lights out!" I ordered. I connected the lamp and turned it on.

Simon plunged the room into darkness. The only light was the blue light from the Wood's lamp.

I opened the trash can and shone the light inside. The towel lit up with bright green patches.

"It's anti-freeze! It always lights up with Wood's light!" I shouted.

Simon turned the lights back on.

"But it was the cat's urine!" he pointed out.

"Yes, but how did the cat get anti-freeze? Because Ulysses was drinking it and the cat licked it after Ulysses collapsed. Anti-freeze smells sweet, so the cat licked it too!" I guessed.

"I don't know if St. Paul's will buy that," Simon said, quietly.

I had no option. Minutes later, I was on the phone with the ER at St. Paul's in Fort Worth.

"Well, I need to fill out this transfer form," the transfer coordinator said, bored.

"I've already given you all his information," I said.

"Wait," he said.

There was silence.

"Wait," he repeated.

I waited.

"Your call is very important to us," a voice said. "Please continue to hold."

I waited several minutes.

"Hello?" I ventured.

"Your call is very important to us," the voice assured me. "Please continue to hold."

I waited. The coordinator returned.

"Okay, I'm almost done. We got one deal left. What was the diagnostic test you guys did?" the transfer coordinator asked.

"What do you mean?" I asked, my mouth drying up.

"The *test* by which you are *sure* that's the poison, that's why we call it a *diagnostic test*," the coordinator said, sarcastically.

I hesitated.

"Surely you've done *something* to confirm the poison?" he asked. "In your little po-dunk hospital?"

"Yes!" I declared, and looked at Simon for an answer. He threw his hands up and shook his head in despair. He pointed to the cat and shone the Woods light on the cat. Bright green spots appeared on its legs.

"What, exactly, was the confirmatory test?" the coordinator demanded.

"A positive cat scan," I stated, calmly.

There was a pause.

Simon suppressed a guffaw. He covered his face with his hands.

I froze.

"What did you say?" the coordinator asked again.

"A positive cat scan," I repeated, with authority.

"A positive CAT scan," the coordinator repeated.

He paused. I looked at Simon and shrugged helplessly.

"Okay, fine. Send him over!" the coordinator said, without

enthusiasm.

"Thank you!" I said, calmly.

I put the phone down and jumped with joy.

"So what are you doing for poor Mr. Ulysses?" Jane asked, as I left. She had the recorder in her hand, "Is he going to be left to die here?"

"Not at all. I have spoken to the Emergency Room at St. Paul's in Fort Worth, and they have accepted him."

"What was wrong with him?" she persisted.

"I can't reveal that," I said. "Patient confidentiality. I'm surprised you don't know about patient confidentiality."

She glared and switched off the tape recorder.

"Off the record?" she queried.

"I'm sorry. You can turn your other recorder off now," I said, sharply.

Jane Pettenguard was taken aback, but recovered and attacked.

"You were lying to the hospital in Fort Worth, I'm sure of it! They never accept patients easily. How did you convince them? You must have lied!"

"I took care of the patient to the best of my ability, with whatever resources I had," I said.

"My readers have a right to know what you did! They have a right to know what's going on in this strange little hospital with a British doctor and British nurse!"

"Indian doctor and British nurse," I corrected.

"My readers want to know what really happened to the Woodcox boy, the Woodcox boy!"

I walked past her.

"Tell your readers you've been recording them secretly for years with a recorder that looks like a hearing aid. They have a right to know what you did!" I said as I pushed past the ER doors.

"Did you lie to get your patient transferred?" Jane called out.

I shook my head and went out to the parking lot.

I was merely being economical with the truth, I thought to myself.

CHAPTER 12

THE GIFTS OF CHRISTMAS

It was ten o'clock in the morning on Christmas Day and I was in the hospital, ready to make rounds. I pushed the cart out of the nurses' station and checked the three charts in it. Ruth Ann, the head nurse, emerged from the break room with a brightly wrapped gift. I imagined a bottle of whisky as she set it down carefully.

"I'm ready!" she declared. "I'm just going to sit this doo-dad here. A gift for you!"

"A gift for me? From you?" I asked.

She looked hesitant.

"Actually, it's a gift from all of us," she said, waving at the other nurses, who looked embarrassed.

I was taken aback.

"That's very thoughtful!" I said. "I'm sorry, I don't have a gift for you and the staff. At least, not right now."

She shook her head.

"Oh, it's nothing, really! It's just a small something. Let's start rounds," she said, and hurriedly collected a clipboard, notepaper and the medication logs.

I lifted the gift and shook it gently.

"It seems to be a bottle of some liquid," I observed. "Is it wine?"

Ruth Ann turned red and shook her head.

"Oh no, Doctor! I would never touch alcohol!" she declared.

"I'm curious. May I open it?" I asked.

Ruth Ann hesitated.

"It's your gift," she shrugged.

I paused.

"Perhaps I should wait until after rounds," I said.

"Okay, then," she said, briskly, and pushed the cart towards a patient's room. She seemed relieved.

"No, I've changed my mind. I'm going to open it right now," I said.

It was reassuringly heavy. I tossed the golden bow and ripped off the blue wrapping. It was, indeed, a bottle of liquid, and it was *partly* alcohol.

"Mouthwash!" I said, in disbelief.

"Yes!" Ruth Ann mumbled.

"Mouthwash?" I repeated, feeling shocked and insulted.

"You know how you love them pickled onions and okra and raw onions on your food in the hospital cafeteria?" she explained earnestly.

"Are you saying, my mouth smells?" I asked, incredulous.

I stood still and demanded an answer.

"Yes, it does! Ask anyone!" she said, flatly.

I was horrified.

"So I've been walking around, talking to you and the staff and all the patients and all along I've had bad breath?" I asked, numbed.

"Yes. But not *that* bad," she admitted. "I mean, I've smelled worse."

"That doesn't make me feel any better."

Ruth Ann nodded towards the patient's door.

"Can we start? It's Christmas and I want to go home," she said.

"I'm just getting over your gift. It was unexpected. Unusual gift, if I may say so," I sniffed.

"Think of it as frankincense or myrrh," she said, brightly.

We saw the first patient. As we emerged from the room, the clerk, Helga Hunnicut, called out.

"Doc, it's your wife! Want me to take a message?" She asked.

"No, I'll talk to her right now," I said. I went back to the nurses station.

Maya was worried.

"I hate calling you in the hospital, but I'm really worried. Priya and Anjali went to the Hastings' house this morning. Brooke wanted to show them her presents. Brooke was trying to show them a video on that big TV they have in the den. The thing fell on her!"

"What?" I jumped.

"The big TV *fell* on Brooke! It hit her on the head. Luckily, there were plenty of adults nearby. They got her out. She was pretty dazed. There's a little swelling of her forehead. They're watching her at home. But Priya says Brooke can't see properly now!"

"That's not good! There could be a serious head injury," I said.

"So what should I tell them?" Maya asked.

"Tell them to come to the ER right away. I'm on call. I'll be done with rounds by the time she gets here. I need to take a look," I said.

"Do you think it's serious? The parents were a little reluctant because she looks okay, and they've got a lot of family over," Maya explained.

"I understand," I said, "but I really need to see her. This could be something very serious. Tell them to bring her. I'll wait here."

I hung up.

"So you couldn't wait? You opened your gift?" Helga

chuckled.

"Yes," I admitted.

"We were all kind of embarrassed, but Ruth Ann said you would understand," Helga said.

"I'm not embarrassed. I'm mortified," I said.

Cherie giggled.

"Well, we're only trying to help. Remember the time you came to the hospital with lip balm on your lips?"

I nodded, wearily. I really didn't want to hear it again.

"Only it was glitter glue! We couldn't stop laughing!" Helga guffawed.

"I'm going to resume rounds," I said, trying to maintain my dignity. "I'm expecting a young girl, Brooke Hastings, eight years old, in the ER, with a head injury."

"I'll call the ER and let Simon know," Helga said.

"Thank you."

"Dr. Mathur, let me know what you think about the mouth wash. I want to use it for my Freddie," she said, smiling.

"Your boyfriend?" I asked.

She shook her head.

"My dog," she replied. "His breath smells *so* bad!"

I examined Brooke in the ER. She was a wisp of a girl, pale and blonde, her braided hair pulled back and pinned. She wore a red velvet dress, white leggings, and a peppermint bow. She rocked her legs back and forth and twisted her body repeatedly. She rubbed her forehead.

"Hello Brooke! Merry Christmas!" I said.

Brooke jumped. She said nothing.

"I know you don't want to be here, do you, Brooke?" I asked as I approached.

Her mother stepped up. She was a petite brunette.

"Dr. Sandi, thank you for seeing her," she said. "But I'm sure it's only a bruise. Nothing worse."

"Holly, I agree there may be nothing wrong with Brooke, but that looks like a pretty big lump on her forehead."

"Thank you for seeing her," she said. "Hugh will be here PDQ. He's making arrangements for all our guests. We have a lot of family over."

I examined Brooke. There was a blue lump the size of a lollipop above her left eye. She stiffened as I examined her.

"It doesn't hurt, Mr. Mathur," she said earnestly. "Really, it doesn't."

"She was changing the channels or something on the big TV in the living room," Holly explained. "It's always been kind of wobbly. Guess it fell on her. I heard this big crash and came running. Brooke was hit on the side of her forehead and knocked down. Lucky she wasn't smushed underneath it!"

"Thank goodness for that!" I said.

I read her ER record. Brooke Hastings, eight years old, resident of 618 High Road, Hotspur, no medical history of note, on no medicines and with no drug allergies. No surgeries in the past.

"Brooke, you know me. I'm Priya and Anjali's dad," I said, calmly.

Brooke nodded warily.

"I'm just going to examine you a little more. It's not going to hurt, okay?"

Brooke nodded, slowly.

"I'm going to shine a light in your eyes first from the right and then from the left. Just look straight ahead."

Her left pupil did not respond to the light. I turned off the flashlight.

"Okay, now I want you to look at the bulb of this flashlight and focus on the tip of the bulb. I'm going to bring it closer and closer. You just keep looking at the top of the bulb."

Her left pupil did not respond. I pointed to the eye chart on the opposite wall.

"I want you to cover your right eye and read the smallest letters you can."

She covered her right eye and squinted at the eye chart.

"I want you to cover your right eye and read these letters with your left eye," I said, and removed an IV pole parked in front of the eye chart.

"Why?" she looked up and asked.

"Because it tells me if the inside lining of your left eye is working," I explained.

"Okay," she shrugged. She read down to the last line.

"Very good! Now do the same thing with the other side."

Brooke read down to the last line with her right eye as well.

"Now I'm going to shine a light in your eyes again. Look straight in front, at the door behind me."

"Why are you doing that?" she asked again.

"When I shine a bright light in your eye, too much light goes in and a nerve narrows the opening to protect the eye from too much light. The opening is that black dot in the center of the eye. When there's too much light, like when I flash a light into it, the black spot should become smaller to keep the extra light out."

"What if there's too little light?" Brooke asked.

"Then the opposite thing should happen. The black spot should become bigger, to let more light in, to help see in the darkness."

"So you want to see if that nerve is working?" she asked, brightly.

"Exactly! You're a smart young lady!" I said.

Brooke beamed.

I examined the right side first.

"Now the other side. Look at the door again."

The right pupil constricted, but the left one did not.

"Now I want you to look at the tip of my pen," I said, holding it up, "and keep looking at it. But don't move your head, just follow it with your eyes."

"Okay," she said, cautiously.

She faltered as I went from left to right.

"It gets blurry," she said.

"Did you see double?"

"Yes."

"Do you see double when you look to the right or the left or both?"

"Only when I look to the right."

"I need to look at the inner lining of your eye, the retina. So I'm going to look with a very bright light," I explained, "and I'm going to be very close to your face."

I examined her with an ophthalmoscope. Her retinas were normal.

"Your breath smells funny," she giggled.

I thought of the mouthwash and shuddered.

"Brooke!" her mother scolded. "That's not how you talk to the doctor!"

I continued my neurological exam. I checked for sensation, tone, movements, coordination and gait. Everything else was normal. I ran my fingers over the big blue bump on her forehead. It seemed a little bigger.

Her father, Hugh Hastings, burst in. He was the local insurance agent, a tall well-built man with a middle parting and a penchant for bowties.

"Is everything okay?" he asked, breathlessly.

"Give me a few minutes," I said.

I listened to her heart and lungs and palpated her abdomen. I looked over her arms and legs for a rash.

"Is everything okay?" her mother repeated, worried.

"Well, *almost* everything's okay. Holly, Hugh, I have to tell you, I'm worried about her left eye. It's not moving properly and the eye reflex isn't good."

"So what does that mean?" Holly asked.

I hesitated.

"I think we need an urgent CT scan of the head. I'm worried there could be something damaging the nerve that goes to the left eye," I explained.

"But she can see just fine," Holly protested. "You just checked her!"

"Yes, but she isn't able to move her left eye properly."

"Could it just be bruised?" Holly asked.

"Yes, possibly. But the critical thing is, the pupil of the eye – the black spot in the middle – does not respond to light. It should become smaller when I flood the eye with light, but it doesn't."

"Really?" Holly sounded unconvinced.

"Really. I checked twice," I replied, firmly.

She looked at her husband. He shrugged.

"Would you like me to show you?" I asked.

"Would you mind?" Holly said. "I don't want to make you mad at me. I'm not doubting you."

I smiled.

"Hugh, come closer. I want you to see this as well," I said.

Hugh sidled up and stood behind Holly.

"Watch the black spot in the middle of the right eye. I'm going to shine a bright light on the right eye first. The black spot will get smaller."

We watched the right pupil rapidly constrict with light.

"Now watch this," I said, and repeated the exercise.

The left pupil responded sluggishly.

"It responded!" Holly cried. "I saw it!"

"Yeah! It got smaller! I saw it too!" Hugh whooped.

I sighed.

"It did get smaller, but very slowly. It's *not* normal. I've seen this many times. This is *not* the normal reaction," I insisted.

"She responded, Doc!" Hugh declared. "That's good news, right?"

"Yes, but it was very slow! It was not normal!" I persisted.

Hugh crossed his arms and stepped back.

"Seems to me, her eyes are okay. Doc, you sure about this deal?" he asked, shaking his head.

"Yes, I'm sure. This is abnormal and she needs to go to a children's hospital to get a CT scan of her head and see a neurosurgeon," I said, my voice rising.

"Doc, I know you don't like us questioning you, we don't doubt you, just don't know we really need a second opinion, you know," he went on.

Holly pulled back and shook her head.

"I'm really worried, Hugh," she interjected.

"So am I, honey, but she just got a little bump and now we are talking about going out of town!" Hugh turned to me, "Don't tell me we need an ambulance?"

"Hugh, she needs to go to the Children's Hospital in Fort Worth, right away. I think there's a bleed inside her skull, and it could cause some serious brain damage!"

Hugh threw his hands in the air.

"You think? You *think*? Doc, I got all the respect in the world for you, you're a great guy and all, but you gotta do better than that!" Hugh looked at Holly for support.

Holly put her hands on her hips and shook her head.

"Hugh, I'm really worried," she said, quietly.

"About what, honey? She looks fine to me," Hugh said.

"I don't know. Something, I don't know what," Holly replied.

They looked at me.

"Doc, are you really sure there's something serious? She looks okay other than that shiner, and I've had 'em a lot worse than that!" Hugh chuckled.

I thought before I answered.

"I really think there's a serious problem. In fact, I think it's so serious I think we need to get a helicopter and fly her to Fort Worth. Right away!"

Hugh took a step back and shook his head.

"*Whoa! Whoa!* Whoa there! A helicopter?" he was astonished.

"Yes."

"You gotta be kidding me! A helicopter for a shiner? A helicopter?"

"I think she really needs it," I insisted.

Hugh turned to Holly, incredulous.

"Hugh, I think we gotta do what the Doc says," she said, quietly.

"Do you know the cost of those things?" Hugh exploded. "Do you? Take a guess!"

Holly shrugged.

"Five to ten thousand dollars! Five to ten *thousand!*" he cried. "We don't have that kind of money to burn!"

Brooke began to cry. Her parents rushed to her side and hugged her.

"It doesn't matter. We've got good insurance. I'm sure they will cover it," Holly said, stroking Brooke's face.

"Only if it's a medical emergency," Hugh retorted. "If we

get there and there's nothing wrong, then they won't cover it."

He looked at me in panic.

"I can get her there real fast! I can get a police car with a siren and go a hundred miles an hour!" he pleaded.

"It won't be safe. The weather's been terrible. We've just had that terrible dust-storm and there's another thunderstorm coming in from Dallas."

"I promise I will get her there in three hours! There's no traffic, it's Christmas!"

"But if we have a problem on the road then we're really stuck," Holly pointed out. "There's hardly anyone to help, everyone's home for Christmas."

Hugh looked at her in astonishment.

"Are you kidding me? Are you seriously kidding me? Are you saying we should get a chopper?"

"Hugh, I know it's a huge expense, but it's the safest thing to do. We're just too far away and we don't have those specialists in Abilene. We've got to get her to Children's in the metroplex!" I insisted.

Hugh shook his head and sat down on the gurney next to Brooke. He pointed to me.

"You dang sure about this?" Hugh demanded.

"No," I admitted.

"You're not sure? And you really want us to possibly pay ten thousand bucks for a joy ride just because you *thought* so?" Hugh asked, angrily.

"We got to do this, Hugh," Holly whispered.

Hugh slumped.

There was silence, except for Brooke's sniffing.

Then Hugh spoke.

"Okay, Doc. Go for it! Get the dang helicopter!"

I returned home thirty minutes later. Priya was there at the door.

"What happened to Brooke?" Priya asked, immediately.

"She hurt her head. I sent her to see a specialist in Fort Worth," I replied.

"You smell funny," Priya noticed. "Did you just brush your teeth?"

"No," I answered, "mouthwash."

"Did she go with her mom and dad?" Priya asked.

"No, she went by helicopter. Her mom and dad are driving there as fast as they can in their car," I said.

"Why did she go in a helicopter?" Priya questioned.

"She needed to go to a big hospital very quickly," I explained.

"Did her mother go with her?" Priya asked.

"Brooke's parents couldn't fit in the helicopter because it was full of medical people and machines, so they got in their car and they're driving to the hospital," I answered.

"Come on, sit down!" Maya said. "We haven't eaten. We've been waiting for you."

Maya had prepared buttery tomato spaghetti and turkey meatballs. She added breadcrumbs to the pasta, and spooned sour cream over it. I laced my food with red pepper flakes and listened to Priya describe the scene at the Hastings house.

"That crash was so loud! And then Brooke screamed, and her mother screamed and her dad came running and he called his brother and they lifted the TV off Brooke. There was glass everywhere but it didn't cut Brooke's face and Brooke had a big swelling on her head and it looked blue and when I was standing next to her she didn't even see me even though I was standing *right* next to her!"

Anjali put down her fork and nodded grimly, then went back to eating.

"I said to Brooke, Brooke, *Brooke*, are you okay, and she

didn't answer and so I asked her again and she still didn't answer!" Priya continued.

"Eat your dinner, Priya," Maya said.

Priya swallowed an entire meatball.

"She didn't even say anything! She just sat there and started crying. She could see Anjali who was in front of her but not me!" Priya went on.

"You were standing on her right side?" I asked.

"I'm not sure, maybe. She didn't talk to me or her dad, she just cried and cried, then her mommy gave her some water and she stopped and they made her lie down and her mommy said should we take her to the hospital and I called mom and *she* said they should take her to the hospital and so I told them," Priya continued, breathlessly.

"Daddy!" Anjali spoke up.

"Is she really sick?" Priya asked, urgently.

"Daddy!" Anjali repeated.

"Is she going to die?" Priya asked, tears welling up.

"Daddy!" Anjali repeated, wearily.

"Hang on, Priya. Let me talk to Anjali. What's up, Anjali?"

Anjali appeared flustered.

"Brooke is sick? Really?" she questioned.

"Yes, I think so."

"That's why Daddy sent her in a helicopter!" Priya explained. "She's really sick! She could die! On Christmas!"

I didn't contradict Priya. Anjali was stunned.

"Is that really true?" Maya asked. "Or are you just being a little dramatic?"

I hesitated.

"Well, I think it's very serious. She couldn't move her left eye properly. I mean, she had some control, but there was definitely loss of movement. Her pupil didn't respond properly to light. She could have an internal bleed inside the skull. The danger is, blood inside the skull squishes the brain against the bone and crushes it, and it can cause brain damage," I explained.

"But a helicopter? Isn't that a little excessive?" Maya asked.

I sighed.

"I don't know. It's expensive, yes, but brain damage can happen in minutes and can be irreversible," I said, toying with my food.

"Not just expensive, *very* expensive. I heard that the bill can easily be ten or fifteen thousand dollars," Maya said.

"True. But the Hastingss have insurance," I countered.

"Yes, but the insurance will only pay if they agree it was medically necessary. If the insurance company decides it wasn't medically necessary, then they can refuse to pay for the helicopter," Maya pointed out. "So I really hope you know what you're doing."

"How do you know all this?" I asked, in wonder.

"Mrs. Templar called and told me. She knew everything that was going on," Maya answered.

"No secrets in this town," I observed.

"None at all. Now let's go and see the Christmas movie you bought for the girls. Which one did you get?" Maya said.

"I bought *Gandhi*," I said, proudly. "It won several awards and it's about India. Good for the girls to know something about India. It's going to be a great Christmas gift for them."

Maya looked doubtful.

We took a bowl of popcorn and went to the bedroom. Maya sank into the recliner and I lay down with Priya and Anjali on either side. I pulled them in closer to me.

We had just started watching when the phone rang. Maya paused the movie. Gandhi froze in South Africa.

"Doc, this is Nancy Abernaty! I'm the pilot of the

helicopter that just picked up your patient, Brooke Hastings."

"Go ahead."

"Can you hear me?"

"Not clearly but good enough," I answered.

"Your hospital patched me through. Hey, listen, there's real bad fog in Dallas. I can do an instrument landing but it's risky. I recommend we divert to Wichita Falls. They got a CT brain scanner there," Nancy blared over the din.

"I understand, but Brooke needs a CT and a neurosurgeon. They don't have a neurosurgeon in Wichita Falls," I said.

"Doc, her vitals are stable, and her neuro signs are stable. It's risky to land in Fort Worth. Do I have your permission to divert to Wichita Falls?" Nancy had to yell.

There was a loud whine like a cloth blocking a vacuum cleaner.

I thought quickly.

"No! Do not divert! She needs to go to Fort Worth!" I insisted.

"Her neuro signs are normal! I repeat, her neuro signs are normal! May we divert?" her voice boomed over the noise.

"No! No! Don't divert! Just land somewhere safe and get an ambulance!" I yelled back.

"Doc, the landing is dangerous! I cannot jeopardize everyone on board! I need your permission to divert!" Nancy repeated.

"No! Do not go to Wichita Falls! Just land anywhere nearby that's safe and take the patient by ambulance the rest of the way!" I raised my voice, and gripped the phone tightly. "Listen to me! Do not divert! Do not divert!"

There was a short pause.

"Hold on, Doc! I'm going to talk to my medical director!"

"No, wait! This is my patient! Your director can't overrule

me! She needs to go to Fort Worth!"

I sat up in bed and blared.

"Do not divert! Do *not* divert!"

But the line went dead.

I called the hospital.

"I need to speak to the helicopter pilot," I said, controlling my voice. "It's very urgent! Reconnect me ASAP!"

"Let me try," the operator said, calmly.

I waited. The girls sat up and looked at Maya, who shrugged.

"I can't get through, Dr. Mathur," the operator said, finally.

"Try again," I ordered. "I really need to speak to the pilot."

"I've tried four times already. I'm not getting through. They were headed into a storm."

"Okay, try their head office in Lubbock. Maybe they can patch me through."

"Dr. Mathur, don't fret yourself. I'm going to call them and I will call you back," the operator said. "I promise."

I hung up and waited a few minutes.

No phone call.

Maya started the movie.

Gandhi organized a movement in South Africa to resist the British. A peaceful protest was broken up by the police, who beat the protesters mercilessly. Gandhi was beaten and jailed.

The phone rang.

"Doctor, no one can get through. The Lubbock office says there's bad weather and they've lost touch with the helicopter. They said it happens, not to get too worried. They're going to keep trying, and they know you want to talk to the pilot," the operator relayed.

"Please tell the office that the patient must go to Fort Worth, not Wichita Falls," I said.

"The office said their medical director overruled you and

told them to go to Wichita Falls," the operator said. "They are contacting Wichita Falls Regional Hospital."

I slammed the phone down in anger. The girls looked at each other and remained silent.

After a few minutes, we returned to the movie. Gandhi returned to India. There was famine in Bengal, and the British did nothing to help. Millions starved. Gandhi went to Bengal and organized protests and was arrested again.

The girls started covered their faces with the blanket, and peeped out after a few minutes.

"This is too sad," Maya announced.

"Well, this is all true," I countered.

"Who wants to come with me and get some hot chocolate?" Maya asked.

Anjali scrambled out hastily and shot off. Priya snuggled closer.

"Are they still hurting him?" she asked, looking up at me.

"No," I smiled. "You can watch again."

But Gandhi's ordeals had just begun. There were more riots, a police station was burned down, the British flogged men and women refusing to pay a tax on salt, and there was a massacre of people who had gathered to hear a pro-independence speaker. Men, women and children were cut down by machine-gun fire. It was horrific. Priya burst into tears and I struggled to hold back my own. She bolted under the covers again and refused to come out. I reached for the remote, but the phone rang.

"Dr. Mathur?" the line was clear again.

"Yes," I answered.

"This is Dr. Ballmer at Children's Hospital. I'm a neurosurgeon, and I'm looking after your patient, Brooke Hastings."

"I'm so glad she made it to Fort Worth! I was afraid they were going to divert to Wichita Falls," I said.

"They did," Dr. Ballmer said drily. "Then Brooke had a seizure."

"She had a seizure?" I said.

"Yes. Luckily, they hadn't gone far so they came back. We got her in CT and then to the OR."

"The OR? She needed surgery?"

"Certainly! She had a significant bleed! It was in the left orbit and left frontal lobe."

A wave of shock and relief swept over me.

"I'm so glad she made it there," I said, hoarsely. "Did she do well with the surgery?"

"She's still in the OR. We drained off a lot of blood. The brain tissue was still intact, luckily enough. My junior's closing up. She had a nasty subdural hematoma."

"How big was the bleed?"

"Pretty substantial. The third nerve was compressed and the frontal lobe was full of blood, but, like I said, we drained it off."

"Is she going to be okay? No long term damage?"

"Can't say, it's too soon. But it looks good right now. She's so young, just a little kid. They usually do well."

I exhaled.

"Thanks so much for calling. I was really worried about her."

"Of course! You're welcome. Sweet kid, great case!"

She hung up.

I paused to think. I remembered the swelling around the eye, then the reduced movements of the eyeball, and the sluggish response of the pupil to light. They were all subtle, but they were *there*. And in a young girl in excellent health those minor changes were extremely significant.

I thought about Mr. Rutherford, who had Anjalilar features, but his deficits were explained by diabetes. He had a different pattern: his pupil had been spared.

I remembered medical school in India where my friend Syed had pointed out this difference. *In a third nerve paralysis, if the pupil is spared, then the problem is in the blood supply or diabetes, but when the pupil is also paralyzed, then the nerve is physically damaged.*

Priya peered over the blanket with one eye.

"Is it over?" she asked.

"I think so," I replied.

She sat up and we watched together. Gandhi travelled to London, negotiated with the British and struggled with Jinnah to prevent the break-up of the country. He was unsuccessful, and Britain separated the country into Hindu-majority India and Muslim-majority Pakistan. The separation, called Partition, was the last administrative action of the British and was an epic disaster. The horrors of Partition exploded on the screen. Communities that had lived together for centuries were suddenly ripped apart. People fled with whatever they could snatch, and with fear and anger in their hearts. There was widespread slaughter on both sides.

Priya howled at the sight of blood and spun back under the covers. I watched on, grimly. Priya wailed and whimpered as the carnage continued.

Maya and Anjali marched in with hot chocolate and fresh cookies. Maya turned off the TV and Priya emerged. We sat in silence for a few minutes, trying to forget the movie. Priya struggled at first, then wiped her tears and ate chocolate chip cookies with increasing enthusiasm.

"Brooke's doctor called me," I announced. "She's going to

be fine."

Priya and Anjali perked up immediately.

"So did she need surgery after all?" Maya asked.

"Yes. There was bleeding in the brain," I answered, trying to speak calmly.

Maya nodded.

"She okay?" Anjali questioned.

"Yes," I croaked.

Anjali leapt over Priya and threw her arms around my neck.

"Yes, yes! She's going to be okay!" Anjali exulted.

I found it hard to speak calmly.

"Let's go to the kitchen and make more cookies!" Maya said.

We whooped and ran.

Later that night, Priya and Anjali were lying down in their beds and the house was dark. Maya and I sat on the floor just outside their room, listening to them whisper, ordering them to be quiet and suppressing their chatter.

"I don't think you should have given them so much chocolate!" I hissed.

"I don't think you should have shown them *Gandhi!*" Maya countered. "It made them so sad!"

"It's a great movie!" I protested.

"Yes, but there's a time and a place for everything. And Christmas night is not the time to show your two little daughters *Gandhi*."

I thought about that. The scenes flashed across my mind.

"I guess you're right," I admitted. "It was pretty intense."

"Uh-huh."

There was silence as we waited for the girls to fall asleep. The room lit up as cars passed by, and we saw the outlines of our daughters move restlessly.

"*Gandhi!*" Maya muttered and shook her head. "I can't believe you made them watch it. On Christmas night!"

I smiled at the memory and threw an arm around her shoulders.

"So what was *your* gift for the girls, oh wise one?" I asked.

"Money," she answered. "Now they can go to the post-Christmas sales and buy exactly what they want. No strings attached."

I thought about that. The first two gifts, mouthwash and *Gandhi*, were well meaning gifts but were basically unsolicited advice. They were all about the donor.

The third gift was money. Money, no strings attached.

Freedom, the best gift of all.

CHAPTER 13

THE CATTLEWOMEN'S BALL

Maya called me in the hospital.

"How much longer before you finish?" she asked.

"Not much longer. Should be done in another thirty minutes."

"What happened? You left over an hour ago. I thought you had only three patients in the hospital."

"One of them has a pretty serious heart problem. I'm running some tests."

"Then is it safe to keep the patient here? Should you not send the patient to Abilene or San Angelo? Do what's best for the patient."

"I will, if I can't get the heart rhythm regulated. All she needs is some potassium and she should be fine. Don't need to ship her for something that simple."

Maya paused.

"Are you ready for the Ball?" she asked.

"I'm already wearing jeans and the boots the hospital gave me last year."

"Black shirt and hat?"

"Black shirt, yes. Hat, no. Hat's too big. I look like a garden gnome."

"I want you to be comfortable and enjoy yourself," Maya said. "You get tense in these dances."

"Because I don't know how to dance," I explained, tersely.

"Don't worry. I don't know either. Our accountant, Truett, said he would show us the two-step," Maya said.

"I need time to figure it out," I grumbled. "I can't just pick it up."

"It's the two-step. Two steps! It's not brain surgery!" Maya protested.

"Okay, I'm going to try. I'll get the potassium going on my patient and come pick you up."

I returned home thirty minutes later. I tried on my black Stetson but decided to abandon it. I walked through the corridor to our bedroom. Maya was wearing a denim skirt and white shirt with a tasseled red leather jacket and matching boots.

"Mrs. Rutherford came over that night and brought me the red jacket and boots!" she told me.

"That was really nice of her to make that long drive in the dark," I said.

"Mrs. Priestley is already here at home. The girls adore her. She makes cookies with them, then they draw and color, then she reads stories," Maya said.

"And very little TV," I added.

"Exactly," Maya nodded.

I went and said goodbye to the girls. They were huddled around the dining table.

"Well! You look like a real cowboy now, Dr. Mathur!" Mrs. Priestley exclaimed. The girls laughed.

"No, he Indian!" Anjali chuckled.

"Will you tell us an Akbar and Birbal story when you come home?" Priya asked.

"If it's not too late. Otherwise, tomorrow," I promised. Mrs. Priestley guided them into the kitchen and started measuring flour and sugar. They were completely absorbed by the prospect of baking cookies. Maya and I crept out.

We drove down the hill and turned on Commercial. We drove past the Woodcox house.

"That house takes up the whole block!" Maya remarked.

"You don't realize it because it's surrounded by trees. But you're right. That house takes up the entire block."

"I heard something terrible happened to them," Maya said.

"Yes."

"But you can't talk about it, I know."

The Cattlewomen's Ball was in the high school auditorium. We pulled into the school parking lot and hunted for a spot. There were two trucks labeled *The Flying Butt-Resses*, with bright images of guitars and dancing cowboys and cowgirls, with arched derrieres. Strains of music serenaded us as we parked and walked up.

"That must be the live music they promised," Maya said.

We were greeted by the Rutherfords and the Templars.

"We're delighted you're here! Maya, you look adorable in that jacket!" Agatha Templar said.

"It's Patty's jacket; she let me borrow it," Maya smiled.

"You can keep it if you like," Patty offered.

"Not at all," Maya said, "but I really appreciate your helping me select it. You have to tell me where you shop."

"The jacket's from Vegas, but you and I are going to go shopping at Neiman's in downtown Dallas. Let's spend some of Sandi's money!" she chortled. "And they have a great restaurant!"

We found our table and sat down. Truett and Mediera Weatherford were seated there. We greeted them and others seated nearby.

"Let me show you the two-step," Truett offered Maya.

He led Maya to the dance floor and asked the band to play a slow number. He showed Maya the steps, and she caught on quickly. She came back excited.

"It's *so* easy! And so much fun!" she exclaimed.

"I hope so," I said, doubtfully.

"Don't worry! Let me show you," Mediera offered. We stood up to start my lesson, but the lights dimmed and the program began. We returned to our seats and sat down.

Patty Rutherford stepped into the spotlight. She welcomed everyone and introduced the band. She led a prayer and then talked about the Cattlewomen's Ball.

"Welcome to the thirty-third Cattlewomen's Ball! We are delighted to have you all here today! I wanted to point out the main purpose of this event: to support the 4-H program and other rural programs for girls. We want to encourage girls to apply for scholarships and learn the cattle business and agriculture, we want them to be the future farmers and ranchers of America," she explained, to enthusiastic applause.

A buffet dinner was served and the lights dimmed further. Maya and Truett and Mediera shot off to the dance floor. I was relieved to have been left alone in the darkness. I finished my strawberry shortcake and then nibbled at Maya's pecan cobbler. I was helping myself to ice cream when I was interrupted.

"Well, Dr. Mathur!" Patty declared. "Here you are, sitting all by yourself! You need to get on the dance floor and cut loose!"

"I'm okay," I mumbled, feigning tremendous interest in the ice cream scoop.

"No, you're not! Get up and start dancing! Forget about the hospital!"

I shook my head and balanced a large spoonful of ice cream.

"Don't tell me, you don't know how to dance?" she asked, incredulous.

I shook my head.

"You're right," I mumbled. "I can't dance."

"Nonsense! So you're sitting here all mopey and sad for yourself!"

"No, I'm enjoying the music," I lied.

She grabbed my hand.

"Come on up. I'm going to teach you myself!" she declared.

"No, I don't want to dance," I protested. "I can't dance!"

"Nonsense!" Patty dismissed my protests and dragged me to the dance floor.

"It's the two-step. You put your arms around me thusly, and just follow my lead."

She started the two-step. I stared down, but couldn't see a thing. It was too dark.

"I can't see your feet!" I complained. "It's dark, and your long skirt covers them!"

The music blared. I broke away from her embrace.

"What?" Patty asked.

"I can't see your feet!" I repeated. "I can't figure it out!"

"What?" Patty repeated. She saw me as a challenge.

I wriggled and tried to break loose. The band switched to a fast beat. Patty gripped my hands and urged me to try again.

"Oh, I love this song! Let's go!" she laughed.

She pulled me onto the floor. I couldn't see a thing, and the music was so loud I couldn't hear Patty. I tried to keep up, but stepped on her feet repeatedly. She winced and hobbled. We started again. I stepped on her feet again. She convulsed and swore. We started all over again.

I decided to plant my steps to her side, to avoid her feet, but she kept twisting so that we would stay aligned. I kept crushing her feet. She began to whimper and wail. I switched to a high-stepping trot to spare her feet. Within minutes of the high stepping gait, I snared the edge of her long skirt and pinned it to the ground. Her body twisted suddenly and she let go of me. She cried out and pitched backwards, her arms flailing.

I watched in horror as she crashed. She had a look of shock, anger and betrayal seared on her face. As she fell, she hit Truett and grasped his shirt. He lost his balance and fell on top of her. I lunged sideways and hit a table.

The crowd gasped. The music stopped and the lights went back on again. I helped Patty up. Truett got up and regarded his shirt. The hall went silent as everyone gaped at the three of us.

"Mediera never ripped my shirt off," he grinned.

Patty was not so forgiving. She marched me back to my table.

"You're right, Dr. Mathur! You *really* don't know how to dance!" she said bitterly.

"I'm so sorry," I said.

Maya came up to us.

"Patty, we apologize. Did you get hurt?" Maya asked.

"I have never, never fallen down on the dance floor! Never in thirty-three years!" she cried.

"I'm so sorry," I repeated, miserably.

Patty stormed off. There was shocked silence.

My face burned and I kept my head down. Finally the lights dimmed and the music resumed. I waited a few minutes then crept outside. Maya found me sitting on the back fender of the Flying ButtResses truck.

There was an announcement that could be heard outside the gym and up and down Commercial Avenue.

"Is there a doctor in the house?" a voice boomed.

There was a pause.

"Is there a doctor in the house? No? Then it's safe to dance again!"

There was a gale of laughter and the music resumed.

A police car in the parking lot flashed its lights at me.

"Doc! All okay? This is Kelly," a voice inquired.

"Everything's okay," Maya replied, and sat next to me.

She draped an arm around my shoulders.

"It's okay. Don't be so upset," she said.

I pulled her arm off.

"It was awful," I admitted.

Maya laughed.

"Yes, you were terrible. What was funny was that you looked so devastated!"

"I made them all fall down!"

"Yes. So what?"

"I looked stupid."

"No, you looked clumsy and confused. How about I show you the steps?"

"No point. It's even darker here."

"Then just dance any way you want."

She stood up and took my hand.

"You don't always have to be the star. It's okay to screw up sometimes," she said.

"I feel small," I said.

"Nobody's perfect."

We heard the music slow down.

"This is a good one," Maya announced. "Let's do this. It's *Waltz Across Texas With You In My Arms*."

I stood up and tried to remember any movie with dancing. I gripped Maya and started to dance.

The police car flashed its lights.

"Don't hop up and down so much, Doc!" Constable Kelly suggested.

"*Everyone's* a critic," I complained.

Maya laughed.

"Maybe you should move from side to side rather than up and down," she suggested.

"This is the stuff they don't teach you in medical school," I muttered. I danced on, doggedly, with Maya in my arms.

We were in a high school parking lot in Hotspur, Texas, smelling a diesel generator and barbecue, waltzing in the black, frigid air, in a vast, open ballroom illuminated by a million glittering stars and a police car.

It was magical.

I stopped by the hospital on the way back. Simon was at the nurses' station.

"Heavens, it's Dr. Rudolf Nureyev, the charming doctor who sweeps women off their feet!" he chortled.

"I can explain," I started.

"I heard you brought the house down!" Simon continued, grinning from ear to ear.

"The lady showing me how to dance fell down," I admitted, trying to sound nonchalant.

"Dragged down the eminent CPA Truett Weatherford and demolished an adjacent table as well!"

"I just bumped into a table! That's an exaggeration!" I protested.

Arabela, the head night shift nurse, returned and clapped her hands. Susan Molinari, another regular of the night shift, joined her.

"I heard about your dancing!" Susan announced gleefully. "You were a disaster!"

I didn't know what to say, so I decided to ignore them all. I opened my patient's chart and checked the potassium level. It had normalized. I slid the chart back into the rack with force. It slid out and fell to the ground. I lunged for it but couldn't catch it. The rack wobbled and Simon steadied it.

"The Doctor hunts down his chart with the effortless elegance of a lion taking down an antelope on the African Serengeti," Simon went on, exaggerating his accent. "The Doctor moves with stealth and brings down his prey suddenly and with great force!"

The nurses cackled with laughter. Susan took pity on me.

"Bless your heart, Doctor," she said. "But why did you start dancing if you're so bad at it?"

I exploded.

"I didn't want to! She made me do it! I told her I *couldn't* do it, and she *insisted* that we do it!"

"So she made you do it?" Susan repeated, unconvinced.

"Yes! She made me do it! I didn't want to do it, and I couldn't keep up with her, it was so dark, and ten minutes later, she fell down with this other guy on top of her!" I stammered.

Simon smiled mischievously. I groaned. I knew exactly what he was going to say.

"That's what the bishop said to the actress!" he quipped.

CHAPTER 14

A BAD STROKE

Three weeks after Christmas, an ice storm descended upon Hotspur. The skies clouded over, the ground hardened and split, and freezing rain fell at night. The rain froze into sheets on the ground and black ice on the roads; the trees, roofs and power lines frosted and dangled opaque daggers and needles. The water glazed the leaves of the live oaks in glassy wafers and hung like pearls from their tips. We heard the stiff branches and leaves crack and shatter whenever the wind picked up. Three gloomy days passed.

Eventually, the skies cleared and the sun returned, but patches of black ice lurked on the roads and sidewalks. The air was so sharp it cut into your breath like a blade. We waited for the afternoons, and only then did we venture out. Priya and Anjali ran into problems immediately.

"I slipped!" Anjali complained.

"There's ice everywhere!" Priya added, "even in the grass! And around the cars and the shed!"

"Did you go on your swing?" Maya asked.

"I tried, but it was so cold! And pieces of ice fell off the branches!" Priya said.

"Do you want to go to the Hastings' house and check on Brooke?" Maya asked.

"Yes! I made a card for her!" Priya was excited. Anjali nodded vigorously.

"Don't take off all your warm clothes, then. Let me call Holly and see if it's okay for us to come over," Maya said.

The phone rang before she could call out. She answered,

and handed it to me, looking puzzled.

"It's for you. It's Mr. Dawkins," she said.

"The administrator?" I asked.

She nodded.

"Hello, David," I said. "What's up?"

"Sandi, we have a problem. Looks like Mrs. Rutherford just had a stroke, like, minutes ago. Her husband just called me. He found her in the barn. He's bringing her right over to the ER."

"David, you know I'm not on call," I said.

"Of course I know that! But our moonlighter didn't show up. Bad roads from Dallas," David explained.

"Don't tell me, it was supposed to be Dr. Ehrlich?" I asked.

David hesitated.

"Yeah. He's the only one we could get. We had already paid his company, Express Medics. They said there was no one else. And we don't have the money to go to another company," David said.

"So we don't have a doctor in the ER?" I said, knowing the answer.

"You got it," David answered, brightly. "You're a genius!"

"Am I obliged to show up? Why not just ship her to Abilene or San Angelo?" I asked, hopefully.

"No you're not *obliged* to do anything. But Mr. Rutherford asked for you. Turns out, he knows you and seems to like you. He gives a lot of money to support the hospital, and he offered to write a letter of support for your green card," David explained.

I considered the situation.

"Wait a minute. She had a stroke! We don't have anything to offer her!" I protested. "If she's really having a stroke then she needs to go to Abilene or San Angelo and get a clot-buster *within the hour!*"

"You mean, streptokinase?" David asked.

"Yes. How do you know that?" I asked.

"Because I was at the Walmart in Brownwood when Robbie Rutherford called. I went to the Brownwood hospital and begged the administrator to release two vials of the stuff and I'm headed to the Hotspur ER right now!" David said, excitedly.

"You're driving?"

"Top speed!"

"That's dangerous!"

"Got me a police escort!" David gloated. "Sirens and all! Man, we're doing ninety!"

"David, there's ice on the roads! Be careful!"

"Just get down to the ER for God's sake! You *got* to do this!" David pleaded.

"I know the Rutherfords," I admitted.

"She's the one you threw down on the dance floor, remember?" David said. "Remember the Cattlewomen's Ball?"

"How could I ever forget?"

"You *owe* her, Doc! She's a good woman, her family's good people! They support the community and especially the hospital!"

I hesitated. The phone call started breaking up.

"And if you help her, old Rutherford's - write you a real nice letter, maybe even - pay for your lawyer!" David's voice came in bursts.

"You're breaking up!" I told him. "Yes, I'll come. See you there."

David had already hung up.

I explained the situation to Maya and the girls. They nodded. Holly invited them over and they prepared to leave.

"You not coming for Brooke?" Anjali asked, irritated.

"No, he's going to the hospital," Priya explained. "Again."

"Mrs. Rutherford's a family friend," Maya explained.

"Brooke is *my* friend!" Anjali retorted.

"I will try to come and join you," I said.

"Promise?" Anjali asked.

"Promise to *try*. Can't promise I'll make it," I answered.

Anjali shrugged on her thick jacket and headed to the door. She didn't wave goodbye.

I parked my Corolla as close to the ER ramp as possible and walked carefully. There was a large white Suburban parked in front of the ramp. It had an R in a circle of barbed wire painted on the side. Simon flung the door open.

"Thanks so much for coming, Dr. Mathur!" he greeted me.

"Glad to help," I answered. We walked briskly.

"Looks pretty bad, if you ask me," Simon went on. "But let me tell you something."

"What?" I asked.

"The husband's a bit, well, *difficult*," Simon said, making a face. "You'll see."

Mrs. Rutherford sat in a wheelchair. The right side of her face drooped and she dabbed the corner of her mouth with her left hand. Her right arm sat limply in her lap. Her white hair was tousled and had straw and mud. Her shirt was soiled and her jeans stained and torn. She smelled of manure and cigarette smoke. She attempted a smile.

"Hurry up, little man! She's had a stroke, damn it!" her husband boomed.

I turned. Mr. Rutherford sat on a stool in the corner, in blue-striped pajamas and bathrobe. He waved impatiently.

"Give her the stuff!" he urged. "Get on with it, man!"

"Let me examine her. I think you're right, but let me check her first," I replied.

Mr. Rutherford shook his head vigorously.

"No! You're wasting precious time! Lord knows how much

time she was there in the barn!"

"Let me talk to her and examine her quickly. Mrs. Rutherford, can you get on the examination table?" I asked. Mr. Rutherford snorted.

She shook her head.

"Can you stand up by yourself?" I asked again.

She shook her head.

"Simon, help me get Mrs. Rutherford on the table," I said.

Simon and I locked the wheelchair and lifted her up gently. There was a sudden fetid smell.

"Good Lord!" Simon exclaimed. "She must have fallen in horse droppings!"

"I don't think that's horse droppings," I said. I recognized the smell.

We settled Mrs. Rutherford down. Her right leg was limp as well.

"Mrs. Rutherford, can you hear me properly?" I started.

She nodded.

"Can you understand what I'm saying?"

She nodded.

"Then look at your husband and blink your eyes," I ordered.

She looked at him and blinked.

"Okay, so you can understand me. Can you tell me what happened?"

She shook her head helplessly.

"Can you tell me anything?" I persisted.

She shook her head.

"How can she tell you anything? She's had a stroke, for crying out loud!" Mr. Rutherford interjected. I ignored him.

"How long had you been in the barn?"

She shook her head.

"We sleep in separate bedrooms," Mr. Rutherford

interrupted, "because I smoke and watch TV late."

"What time does she generally get up?" I asked him.

"Five, four sometimes," he answered.

"When did you discover her?"

"About nine."

"It's nine-forty now, so about forty minutes ago! That means we have only twenty minutes left to give her the streptokinase. That's assuming she had the stroke just before she was discovered. We have to start the medicine within sixty minutes of the stroke."

"You have an amazing grasp of the obvious, little man!" Mr. Rutherford snapped.

I turned to Mr. Rutherford.

"Did she say anything to you?"

Mrs. Rutherford gurgled and finally spoke.

"Shit. Crap," she said with great difficulty, shaking her head in frustration. Tears welled up.

"That's all she can say now," Mr. Rutherford said.

"Shit. Crap," Patty Rutherford repeated, helplessly.

I examined her quickly. The right side of her face didn't move, her right upper and lower limbs were flaccid and she could only say a few words. Her heart rate was rapid and she was pale.

"Mr. Rutherford, she has had a pretty severe stroke. It has damaged the left side of the brain, the part that controls the right side of the body. I know she's right-handed, so that's also bad news. I don't know how long she has been down, but I guess it's much more than an hour."

Mr. Rutherford jumped up angrily.

"Damn it, I don't care! Give her the damn clot buster!" he shouted.

"First of all, I'm not sure whether we're still in time. It's likely the window of opportunity has already gone."

"You don't know that! Your guess is as good as mine!"

"At the very best, there's just a slim chance we are still in time. But there's another problem. She's pale and there's a bad smell about her."

Mr. Rutherford gagged.

"She was in a barn with horses, Doc! What do you expect — French perfume?" he retorted.

"That's not the smell of manure," I said. "That's the smell of blood! She's bleeding internally and it's coming out in her bowel movements!"

"What do you mean?" Mr. Rutherford boomed. "There's no blood!"

"No, I mean, she smells like she's bleeding internally. I think she's passing bloody bowel movements," I explained.

"Ridiculous! She would have told me if she was bleeding!" Mr. Rutherford objected.

"Not if she couldn't speak," I countered.

I turned to Simon.

"I need to do a rectal exam. Get her in a gown, quickly. Get me stat labs, I want a CBC and CMP and a Pro Time. Tell Tom I need the CBC first even before the rest is ready."

"You're going to do a rectal exam?" Mr. Rutherford waddled closer and confronted me. "Are you serious?"

"Mr. Rutherford, I suspect Patty is bleeding internally. She looks pale and she smells like she's passing stools that have blood in them. I have to check her for bleeding, it's very important."

Mr. Rutherford raised his hands and shook his head. He looked at me in astonishment. Then he closed his eyes and calmed himself before continuing to argue.

"No, no, you're not getting this," he protested, speaking slowly and forcefully. "Patty had a *stroke*. She needs the *antidote*, the *blood thinner*, the whatever. That's why we're here. Not for anything else!"

"It's extremely important to figure out if she has internal bleeding, Mr. Rutherford!" I explained. "If she has internal bleeding, we can't give the clot buster!"

"Why the devil not?" he demanded.

"Because the clot buster would make her bleed massively and we won't be able to stop it."

"Then just give her some blood!" Mr. Rutherford cried.

"We only have two units of O negative here. It may not be enough. She could bleed to death!" I explained.

A car screeched to a halt in the parking lot. There were police sirens outside.

"Would you like a type and cross for possible blood transfusion, doctor?" Simon asked, quietly.

"Yes! Keep both units of O negative for her. Mr. Rutherford, I need to do an internal exam on Patty. Would you like to stay here or step out?"

Mr. Rutherford was immobile.

"Where is the damn clot buster? Why are you wasting time?" he repeated, shaking with anger.

We heard footsteps racing up. David Dawkins burst into the room clutching a small icebox. He thrust it into my hands.

"*There!* Give it now, Doc, we got just a few minutes left!" he gasped.

Two deputies jumped in behind him, flushed and breathless.

"He won't give it!" Mr. Rutherford exploded.

David turned to me.

"What do you mean?" he asked, incredulous. "You won't give it?"

I took a deep breath.

"David, give me a minute to examine her. I think she's got internal bleeding," I said.

"So what? Has she had a stroke or not?" David was upset.

"Yes, she's definitely had a stroke. But she smells like she's having internal bleeding. If she has internal bleeding, the clot buster could make the internal bleeding much worse."

"Then give blood! We've got blood!" David argued.

"We only have two units. That won't be enough if she has a bleeding ulcer and we give her streptokinase."

"How much blood does she need?" David answered, his voice rising. "Like, four units? Six? We can get it!"

"No, even that won't be enough, she would just bleed out!" I replied.

"What do you mean, bleed out?" Mr. Rutherford spat.

"I mean, she would bleed to death," I said. "She could bleed to death right here in front of our eyes! In minutes!"

There was a stunned silence.

"You're kidding." David mumbled.

"No, I'm serious."

"She could bleed to death?" Mr Rutherford repeated, in disbelief.

"Yes."

"Before she gets to Abilene or San Angelo?" David asked.

"Yes. She could bleed to death right here," I said, quietly.

David coughed.

"Mr. Rutherford, I have the streptokinase right here, like I promised," he said.

"What good is it?" Mr. Rutherford snarled.

"If you want to sign a waiver, maybe Dr. Mathur can give it to her," David said, helpfully. "Just sign a waiver first."

"A waiver? Saying what?" Mr. Rutherford asked.

"Saying that you understand the risks, but you want to proceed anyway," David explained, smoothly.

I jumped in.

"Wait a minute! I'm not going to approve the streptokinase,

waiver or no waiver!" I said.

"Why the hell not?" Mr. Rutherford bellowed.

"Because it's not in her best medical interest," I said.

"You think I don't know what's best for my Patty?" Mr. Rutherford said.

"I know she's your wife and you love her. But I can't let you force me to make the wrong decision!"

"I don't want her to have a stroke!" Mr. Rutherford bellowed.

"And I don't want her to bleed to death!" I countered.

Mr. Rutherford slammed his hand on the counter.

"You little shit! You useless little shit!" he screamed. David squirmed.

"Mr. Rutherford is quite aware of legal issues. He has often paid for the hospital's lawyers," David said.

Mr. Rutherford struggled to control himself and came forward. He grabbed my hand.

"Doc, I'm releasing you from all liability. All liability! You have no liability for anything! Anything! *Just give her the clot buster!*" he demanded.

I hesitated.

"I am begging you!" he implored. "You'll have no liability! Zero liability!"

"Let me examine her and check the blood count, I'm sure there is internal bleeding," I said.

"We don't have time, Doc!" Mr. Rutherford shrieked.

"Simon! Call Tom! I need that CBC now!"

"Just give the damn medicine!"

"Doc, it's thawed out and ready to go!" David mumbled.

"Give me a second!"

"Doc, give her the medicine! I'm going to sign a waiver and you'll have no responsibility!"

"If she's bleeding, it's completely wrong to give a clot buster, waiver or no waiver!"

Mr. Rutherford grabbed the ampoules out of the icebox and thrust them into my hand.

Simon returned with a slip of paper.

"Hemoglobin's nine!" he announced.

"The hemoglobin's low! She is bleeding!" I cried. I felt vindicated.

Mr. Rutherford shook his head.

"I don't give a rat's ass! Give her this damn medicine and fix the stroke!" he insisted. "Why won't you give it and try it?"

"Because I can put it in but I can't take it out!" I cried.

"What the devil?"

"I can put it in but I can't take it out! Once the medicine goes in, there's no antidote. I can't reverse it. We can't take that risk. We have no backup. And we don't even know when she actually *had* the stroke!"

Mr. Rutherford was dazed.

David leaned forwards.

"Mr. Rutherford has promised to write a letter of support for you to the INS. He will get green cards for you and your family," he said in a stage whisper.

I was upset.

"Everyone get out! I'm going to do a rectal exam."

Simon pushed them out. He helped me turn Patty and we peeled her jeans down. There was an immediate stench.

Her buttocks were smeared with reddish-black tarry feces. I knew immediately that she was bleeding internally. There is a distinctive smell of blood in the bowel movements, an awful stench that every physician knows and dreads.

Simon ripped open a stool testing card. I slipped on gloves and swabbed the material. We placed a sample on the card and added a drop of reagent; it turned dark blue immediately. It was obvious to me, but we wanted to prove there was blood in the stools.

"It's positive, strongly positive," Simon called out.

I called Mr. Rutherford and David back inside.

"It's strongly positive for blood. She is pale and has a low hemoglobin. There's no question now, there's internal bleeding, therefore the streptokinase is completely contra-indicated."

"What do you mean, contra-indicated?" Mr. Rutherford asked.

"We can't give it," Simon announced. "Absolutely the wrong thing to do, sir."

"Give a little and see what happens?" David suggested.

"You can put it in but you can't take it out," Simon repeated.

There was an angry silence.

"You can put it in but you can't take it out?" David repeated blankly.

"That's what the actress said to the bishop," Simon shrugged, desperately attempting humor.

"Shut up!" Mr. Rutherford snapped.

"Just give it, Doc! Please!" David pleaded. He picked up the ampoules and handed them back to me.

"That's eighteen hundred bucks!" he urged.

I looked at them helplessly. Mr. Rutherford turned red and grabbed David by the shoulder violently. David tottered and almost fell down.

"I want her transferred to Abilene *right now!* David, get her there *right now!*" he barked.

"Yes, sir! " he gasped.

"Get us out of this God-forsaken shithole you call a hospital, and away from these damn quacks you call doctors!"

David nodded. Mr. Rutherford pointed at me.

"And you! You smug little shit! I'm going to make sure the

INS kicks your foreign ass out!" he vowed. "I got connections, Doc! You're going to regret this day, regret it big time!"

I didn't know what to say. Mr. Rutherford's face turned purple and he waved his fist. I struggled to keep my voice steady.

"I'm telling you the right thing. We don't know how long she was down before she got here, probably well over an hour, and she's bleeding! There's absolutely no reason to give her streptokinase! It would be completely wrong!" I answered, struggling to contain my anger.

"You came crawling to us when you needed help! And now my wife is going to have a stroke for the rest of her damn life because you, in your damn medical opinion, won't help when she needs it the most!" Mr. Rutherford screamed. He spat on the floor.

"David! Get her out of here!" he yelled and swung out into the corridor.

We heard him in the foyer.

"I will make that doctor pay! I will make this hospital pay!" he raved.

Simon and I silently cleaned Patty. We got her in a patient gown and Simon quickly wiped her face and straightened her hair.

"May I comb your hair, madam?" he asked

Patty nodded. She cried and tried to wipe her eyes with her good hand.

"Shit. Crap!" she repeated.

Simon spoke without looking up.

"I guess we should call the ambulance folks now," he said.

"They're right outside the door!" I mumbled.

The paramedics strapped Patty into their gurney. We copied the lab reports and my notes. Simon called the ER in Abilene and alerted their doctor.

I accompanied Patty to the ambulance and checked her IV and the orders. Simon stuffed her clothes and glasses into a bag and Mr. Rutherford tossed it into the back of his Suburban. He heaved himself into the driver's seat; David clambered into the front passenger seat and they glared at us with cold fury. With the door still open Mr. Rutherford turned to me and made a final announcement. He pointed to me.

"I will *crucify* you!" he swore.

He slammed the door shut. The Suburban shuddered.

The ambulance and the Suburban roared off. Simon and I stood in the parking lot, stunned and silent. My mouth was parched and my legs ached from the tension. A sense of incredible fatigue and failure spread over me. I breathed quickly; the cold, sharp air stung and revived me. I felt terrible and hollow, as if gutted and all hope and happiness had been ripped out. After standing for a few minutes, the numbness wore off and we started feeling painfully cold. We trudged back up the ramp in grim silence.

As we entered the building, Simon spoke.

"Other than *that* little unpleasantness, Mrs. Lincoln, how was the play?"

CHAPTER 15

MEASURE FOR MEASURE

It was bedtime, and Priya and Anjali demanded a new story. They sat upright in their beds, fragrant with rose shampoo and jasmine soap, determined to stay awake.

"Mom put rose water on us!" Priya said, happily.

"Yes, I can smell it. It's wonderful! Are you ready for a story?"

"We've heard all your Akbar and Birbal stories," Priya complained.

"New one!" Anjali demanded.

I closed the blinds and turned out the lights. I pushed the door shut and sat down in the darkness. We could hear Maya cleaning up in the kitchen.

"Have I ever told you a Shakespeare story?" I asked.

"No," Priya said.

"Okay, let's do a Shakespeare story."

"Is it going to be short? You can't make it too short," Priya warned.

"No, in fact they're very long."

"Okay, then. Just so long as it isn't too short," Priya said, warily.

"I promise."

"And it's not sad?"

"No."

"Okay!" Anjali approved.

"Any unicorns?" Priya asked, hopefully.

"No."

I waited, but Priya had no other questions. The story had to be long, have a happy ending, and unicorns were optional.

"Once upon a time, many years ago, in a city called Vienna, there was a man called Claudio," I began. "This man, Claudio, was in love with a girl called Juliet. He wanted to marry her."

"Was she beautiful?" Priya asked.

"Yes, Juliet was very beautiful. She had long black hair like you, and big eyes like Anjali. The king of Vienna had a son called Angelo. The king wanted to see if his son, Angelo, would be a good king. So he said he was going on a holiday for a long time and would come back later, and made his son, Angelo, the king while he was gone."

"So Angelo was the prince?" Priya asked.

"Yes. But he was called Lord Angelo, not Prince Angelo. So the king went away and his son, Lord Angelo, became the king."

"Nice man or bad man?" Anjali asked.

"Lord Angelo was very strict. He was too strict, so he was bad. At that time in Vienna, there was a rule: no one could kiss before they got married. But this man, Claudio, kissed Juliet before they got married, so Lord Angelo put Claudio in jail and said that Claudio would have to die!"

"Die? Why?" Anjali asked.

"Because he kissed her before they were married," Priya explained.

"So the bad Lord Angelo put poor Claudio in jail and said that Claudio must die because he broke the law and kissed Juliet. Claudio said he was sorry and said he was going to marry Juliet anyway but Lord Angelo said no, Claudio broke the law, and had to die."

"That's not fair!" Priya burst out, indignantly.

"No fair!" Anjali echoed.

"Yes, that was cruel. Now Claudio had a sister, Isabella. Isabella was very beautiful and intelligent."

"More beautiful than the first girl, Juliet?" Priya asked.

"Yes."

"Did she have a boyfriend?" Priya wanted to know.

"No, she didn't. In fact, this girl, Isabella, had decided she would *never* have a boyfriend and *never* get married and was just about to join a church and become a nun. Nuns are women who live in the church forever and live like sisters but never get married. They spend all their time working in the church."

"So *she* had never kissed anyone," Priya deduced.

"Right. The very beautiful and intelligent Isabella was the sister of poor Claudio. Poor Claudio was going to die for kissing Juliet before getting married to her. Isabella was very upset at this news and wanted to save her brother. So she went to Lord Angelo and begged him to spare her brother's life."

"Did he listen?" Priya asked.

"Well, Lord Angelo listened to Isabella. And then a funny thing happened. Lord Angelo saw the very beautiful and intelligent Isabella and fell in love with her!"

"*What?*" Anjali was shocked.

"But did the brother die?" Priya asked anxiously.

"Wait. Now Lord Angelo fell in love with Isabella. He wanted to kiss her! But she didn't want to kiss him because she didn't love him. And it was against the law anyway! So she said no to Lord Angelo."

"Good!" Priya said, approvingly.

"And Lord Angelo was already engaged to another woman!" I added.

Both girls gasped.

"*What!*" Priya was outraged.

"*No!*" Anjali protested.

The phone rang in the kitchen and Maya answered it. Priya and Anjali settled down.

"But the bad new king still wanted to kiss the nice girl?" Priya asked.

"Yes," I answered.

"Then they can both be killed!" Priya realized.

"Right! But Lord Angelo was the king so he was okay with breaking the law himself. He told Isabella that if she came to his house at night and kissed him, he would not kill her brother, Claudio."

Priya slapped her headboard angrily.

"That's not fair! He's going to kill the man for kissing but he's going to kiss?" Priya was beside herself. Anjali mumbled in protest. The door opened a crack.

"You have a call. From the ER," Maya whispered.

"Okay, thanks."

"Then what happened?" Priya demanded.

"So the bad Lord Angelo said to Isabella, if you come to my house late tonight and kiss me, I will spare the life of your brother. So now Isabella was stuck! What should she do? Should she kiss Lord Angelo secretly, and that way save her brother? Or follow the law and follow her heart because she wanted to be a nun, and not kiss Lord Angelo? Should she ignore her brother and let him die?"

"No!" Priya cried.

"No fair!" Anjali piped up.

"I have to answer the phone. I'll be right back," I said.

Priya and Anjali were aghast.

"You can't stop *now!*" Priya complained. "That poor man is going to *die!*"

"Don't go, Daddy!" Anjali implored.

"Let me answer. Maybe I won't have to go in."

I walked to the kitchen. I could hear screaming before I put my ear to the phone.

"Simon! What's going on?"

"Dr. Mathur, we've got a young lady, six years old, with a wretched insect in her ear," Simon said.

"It must be alive and trying to move or buzz. That's why she's screaming," I guessed.

"Must feel like a bomb going off every few minutes! What the devil are we going to do?" Simon asked.

"Well, I need to pull it out. But first, lie her down with the bad ear upwards and put in eight big drops of warm oil," I ordered.

"Warm oil? What will that do?" Simon asked.

"It will drown and kill the bug. That will give her some relief and then I'll pull it out."

"We don't have any medical grade oil," Simon said.

"Does she have a perforated or damaged eardrum that the parents know about?" I asked.

"I'll ask them," Simon said.

There was a pause.

"Not that they know of," he relayed.

"Then we can use any oil. Use olive oil or cooking oil, it doesn't matter. Get it from the kitchen or cafeteria, or maybe someone at the nurses station has some. Do it right away! Take that as a phone order! I'm on my way," I said.

I apologized to the girls.

"There's a little girl in the ER and she's six years old. She's really crying a lot so I have to go and see her."

"What about the story?"

"Go to sleep. I'll finish it tomorrow. "

"No, Dad! That's not fair!" Priya complained.

But I was already grabbing my coat and keys and heading out.

Heidi Hernandez was a six-year-old with a blond crew cut and earrings. She was silent and lay curled up on her left side in a fetal position. Her mother and father stood next to her anxiously. The floor had paper towels scattered about and the room smelled of olive oil.

"The oil did the trick! I heated it up in the microwave. She fought me at first and I spilled a lot, but her dad held her down. We got it the second time. I wiped the floor, but be careful, it's slippery. She stopped screaming about two minutes ago," Simon said, relieved.

I greeted the parents and Heidi. I looked at the ER chart. Nothing significant, but she lived on Country Road 808 near the Bloody Basin.

"How did she get a bug in her ear?" I asked.

"I reckon her brothers put bugs in her bed. They're going to get a whipping when I get back!" her father said, grimly.

"She wants to be like them," her mother explained. "Even cuts her hair like them."

"I'm going to deal with them boys," her father muttered.

"You live on CR808, so you must be close to the Rutherford ranch," I said.

"I work for them," her dad said. "Eighteen years."

"How are they doing?" I asked.

"Mrs. Rutherford is back home from the hospital. She had a stroke and a bleeding ulcer. The ulcer got better but she still has a bad stroke. All she can say is shit and crap."

"Mario!" his wife protested.

"What? I'm just telling the doctor what she says."

"And Mr. Rutherford?"

"He's never been the same again. Really upset with the doctors! I think he's never gotten over his son's death and now this!" Mr. Hernandez said, shaking his head.

I looked at Simon.

"I didn't know that they had a son," I admitted. "How old was he?"

"Mid-twenties, I guess. I think he was six or seven when I started working for them, so he must have been twenty-four or twenty-five."

"Were they close?" I asked, knowing the answer.

"Well, when the boy was little, they were real close. He would always hold onto his daddy's legs and he would love on him and they was real close. Later on, daddy and son didn't get along. *Really* didn't get along. I'm talking big fights, screaming fights, throwing stuff. Son finally moved to California."

"What did he die of?"

"DKDC. Don't know, don't care," Mr. Hernandez shrugged. "Boy wasn't a man, he was weird."

"He died of pneumonia, I think," Mrs. Hernandez said.

"Odd thing for a young man to die of," Simon observed. "In my experience, pneumonia usually affects the elderly."

I pondered.

"If Mr. Rutherford was dealing with such a tragedy when his wife had a stroke, that would certainly make him agitated. Did you know that he had a son?" I asked Simon.

"I didn't know either," Simon shrugged. "But it would explain his foul mood. Oh, he was livid!"

My mouth went dry at the memory.

"He threatened to crucify you!" Simon recalled, blithely.

"Thank you for reminding me."

"In case you had forgotten, Doctor."

"I don't think I will ever forget that, Simon."

"*Bloody* awful evening, it was! Man went completely overboard, went bonkers!"

I nodded towards Heidi.

"Let's get that bug out of this little girl's ear."

"Yes, sir!"

"Give me a twenty cc syringe of warm water. Warm but not hot, be careful!"

Simon drew up the sterile water and ran hot water over the body of the syringe for a few minutes. He handed it to me and I approached the little girl. Simon and her mother held her down on her left side, with her right ear pointing towards the ceiling. As I approached, she cried and tried to get up. Her father pinned her down.

"Hold still!" he ordered.

She squirmed again. He gripped her firmly.

"You want to be tough like your brothers? Then you hold still, mi hija!" he ordered.

Heidi whimpered.

"Hold still, mi hija!" her father repeated.

She stopped moving. She sniffed and suppressed a sob.

"No crying!" her father added. "No crying, mi hija!"

She swallowed and became silent.

I placed clean towels around her ear and warned her.

"Heidi, I'm just going to squirt some warm water into your ear. I'm going to do it very slowly," I said.

She didn't answer.

"Go ahead, Doc," her father said.

I held her ear open by pulling upwards and backwards, and gently pushed five cc of warm water into the opening of the ear canal.

"Whoa!" her father yelped. "There's the bug!"

An oval black object had washed out. It was the size of a sunflower seed. I patted it with a dry corner of the towel and peered at it. Mr. Hernandez loosened his grip and Heidi turned to look at the villain.

"Can't tell what kind of bug it is," I admitted. "But I don't think it's the kind that your sons would keep in a bottle."

"How do you know?" Mr. Hernandez asked.

"Too small. Can't hold it between your fingers."

"You're just trying to spare them a whipping," he laughed.

"No, I mean it. Look at the bug!"

"Doc, you got two little girls. Girls are different. We got two boys and I tell you, they would burn the house down if I didn't ride them pretty hard. Boys are different. They need discipline! The rod! That's how a boy becomes a man!"

I plucked an otoscope off the wall.

"I'm going to check her ear canal to make sure it's clear," I said.

Mr. Hernandez turned Heidi's head back down. I looked carefully.

"Looks good. The tympanic membrane is intact," I said.

"What?"

"The eardrum is okay."

"Good. Do you got to do anything else on her?"

"No. We're done. She can go home."

"Doesn't she need some antibiotics?" her mother asked, hopefully.

"Her eardrum looked good, the lining of the canal was good, so, no. No need for antibiotics," I declared.

Heidi's mother looked disappointed.

"Want to give her a shot?" Mr. Hernandez wondered.

"There's no infection. There's no need," I insisted.

Heidi's parents looked at each other and shook their heads.

"She had a bug in her ear!" Mrs. Hernandez protested.

"It didn't damage anything. There's no infection. There's no need for antibiotics," I stood my ground. The parents were sullen.

"You got to give her some antibiotics," Mr. Hernandez tried

again.

"No, she doesn't need them. Her ear looks good, it's not scratched or bleeding and the membrane is fine," I insisted.

I picked up the chart and retired to the dictation room to write.

Mrs. Hernandez spoke in a stage whisper.

"Remember, what Mr. Rutherford said, this is the doctor who doesn't know how to treat anything," she explained.

"Yeah. He don't know how to treat nothing, not stroke, not ear infection, nothing!" her husband agreed.

I wrote a short procedure note. Simon hovered nearby.

"They've gone," he grinned.

"Well, they didn't look too happy when they left," he observed.

"There was no need for antibiotics," I repeated.

"Dr. Ehrlich gives antibiotics like candy," Simon said. "The patients love it."

"Many doctors over-prescribe antibiotics," I said.

"Still, it makes him popular. The ranch hands love to get shots. Maybe you should give shots more often," Simon suggested.

"They're not necessary," I replied.

"But your green card is necessary," Simon countered, "and you need some good letters of support."

I nodded.

"So I should give more shots and prescribe antibiotics even when I don't think they're necessary?" I asked.

Simon shook his head.

"I'm not advocating doing the wrong thing," he said.

"Sounds like it."

"Some rise by sin, and some by virtue fall," Simon declared.

"Shakespeare?" I asked.

Simon nodded.

"Yes. *Measure for Measure.*"

When I returned, the lights were still on. Maya was sitting in the girls' room, braiding Anjali's hair.

"They wouldn't go to sleep. They wanted to hear the rest of your Shakespeare story," Maya explained.

Maya kissed the girls and turned out the lights. Closed the door and settled down on the carpet.

"Okay, so where were we?"

"The bad man had put the good man in jail for kissing his girlfriend," Priya summarized.

"Right. Claudio had kissed his girlfriend and the bad Lord Angelo put him in jail and was going to have him killed."

"You can get *killed* for kissing?" Priya questioned.

"It's just a story. But maybe in the past they did have very cruel punishments for little things," I explained.

"So the bad Lord Angelo wanted to kill poor Claudio, but his sister went to ask Lord Angelo not to kill Claudio!" Priya said.

"Yes. But when Claudio's sister, Isabella, went to see Lord Angelo, Lord Angelo fell in love with her. And you know what he said to Isabella? He said, if you kiss me, I will not kill your brother."

"That's not fair!" Priya burst out again.

"No fair!" Anjali echoed.

"So Isabella was very sad. She didn't know what to do. She didn't love Lord Angelo and didn't want to kiss him. But if she didn't, her brother would die! So she was confused. What should she do?"

"So what *did* she do?" Priya asked, anxiously.

"Now, Lord Angelo actually had a girlfriend. Her name

was something, I can't remember."

"Jasmine," Priya suggested.

"I'm pretty sure it wasn't Jasmine."

"I like Jasmine!" Priya protested.

"Sarah Savannah," Anjali suggested. "I like Sarah Savannah."

"Her name wasn't Sarah Savannah and it wasn't Jasmine. I don't remember. Let's say Helena."

"Why can't it be Jasmine?" Priya persisted.

I sighed.

"Jasmine it is," I conceded.

Anjali whimpered.

"Okay, her name was Jasmine Sarah Savannah. So the mean Lord Angelo said to Isabella, come to my house and kiss me then I won't kill your brother. Isabella was very sad and went to the jail to tell her brother, Claudio. Claudio didn't know what to do. Luckily, the real king, who was in disguise, was pretending to be the priest of the jail. Isabella told him about her problem."

"Did she know that he was really the king?" Priya asked.

"No, she didn't. She thought he was just a holy man who worked in the jail. The king said to Isabella, Isabella, this is what you should do. Agree to meet Lord Angelo, but late at night in the back of the garden, where it's dark. Say that you will not talk. Then send his girlfriend, Jasmine Sarah Savannah, in your place. Then Lord Angelo can kiss his own girlfriend, Jasmine Sarah Savannah, in the dark and will think that he has kissed you!"

"That's a good idea!" Priya nodded.

"I like Jasmine Sarah Savannah," Anjali added, sleepily.

"So Isabella told Lord Angelo that she would meet him in the night, in the back of the garden, and kiss him. So Lord Angelo was very happy and said he wouldn't kill poor Claudio."

"Then what happened?"

"Then that night, Jasmine Sarah Savannah, who was

actually the real girlfriend of Lord Angelo, went to the garden of Lord Angelo where Lord Angelo was waiting. Lord Angelo did not recognize Jasmine Sarah Savannah because it was dark. So he kissed his own girlfriend, Jasmine Sarah Savannah, and thought that he had kissed Isabella."

"He couldn't tell?"

"No. He really thought it was Isabella!"

"His girlfriend didn't say anything?"

"No, she didn't."

"So that he wouldn't know who it was?"

"Exactly."

"Then what did the beautiful nice girl who was the sister do?"

"Later, Isabella told Lord Angelo, remember my brother! You must forgive him now."

"So the brother was freed?" Priya asked.

"No! Lord Angelo changed his mind! Even though he thought Isabella had kissed him, he decided to go ahead and have Claudio killed."

"What!" Priya spluttered in shock.

"Lord Angelo said he wanted Claudio's head cut off and sent to him!"

"*Very* bad man!" Anjali scolded.

"Luckily the real king, who was in disguise, was still at the jail. He convinced the jailer not to kill poor Claudio. Another prisoner had died earlier that morning. He had the jailer cut off the dead man's head and send it to Lord Angelo. He knew Lord Angelo wasn't really going to check."

"Good thing the real king was still there," Priya said. "Otherwise everyone would be so sad!"

"Well, Isabella thought that her brother Claudio was really dead and she became very sad and very angry with Lord Angelo."

"Good thing she didn't kiss him!" Priya said. "I think she should *kick* him!"

Anjali growled in approval.

"Then the real king sent a letter to Lord Angelo telling him to announce that he was coming back and would become the ruler again. He said he would listen to anyone who had a complaint about anything."

"I hope Isabella complained! She should tell him about how mean Lord Angelo was!" Priya interjected.

"So mean!" Anjali agreed.

"The next day the real king returned to Vienna. Everyone still thought that Claudio was dead. Isabella complained that Lord Angelo had promised to spare Claudio if she kissed him, and she did, but Lord Angelo broke his promise and had Claudio killed."

"Actually, Isabella didn't kiss Lord Angelo," Priya whispered.

"You're right!" I said. "Who actually kissed Lord Angelo in his garden in the dark?"

"His own girlfriend, Jasmine!" Priya gloated.

"Jasmine Sarah Savannah!" Anjali corrected.

"Yes. Actually, his own girlfriend, Jasmine Sarah Savannah, had kissed him. Lord Angelo had wanted to do something wrong."

"Did the real king punish Lord Angelo?" Priya asked.

"Lord Angelo told the king that both women were lying."

The girls jumped up in indignation.

"What? No, *he* was lying!"

"Correct. The women said the priest in the jail gave them the idea. So the king said, okay, let's get the priest from the jail. Only, actually *he* was the priest himself. So he said he had to go for some other business and went away. Then he quickly changed into the priest's clothes and came back."

"So did the king tell them all the truth?"

"The real king came back from the jail dressed as a priest. He said, the women are telling the truth and Lord Angelo is lying."

"Yay! Good!" the girls exulted.

"Then the king suddenly took off the priest's disguise and everyone realized that the priest was actually the king!"

"Good! Good!" Priya enthused.

"Then Lord Angelo realized that the king knew everything. So he begged the king to forgive him but also said that he would accept death as his punishment. "

"Good!" Priya said, with less enthusiasm.

"Remember, the king had not yet told Isabella that her brother, Claudio, was alive. Isabella still thought that her brother Claudio was dead. So she was still very sad and very angry with Lord Angelo."

"*Bad* man!" Anjali muttered.

"The king wanted to test Isabella. He asked her if she could forgive Lord Angelo and spare his life or whether she wanted Lord Angelo to die for all the bad things he had done."

"What did Isabella say?" Priya asked, softly.

"Isabella was quiet for some time, then she asked the king to forgive Lord Angelo. She said she was very sad but realized her brother had broken the law against kissing before marriage. She forgave Lord Angelo and asked the king to spare his life."

"That was so nice of her!"

"Yes, it was. The king was very impressed by Isabella's kindness. Actually, *he* had fallen in love with Isabella for being so good."

"So did he marry her?" Priya asked.

"She was nice!" Anjali chimed.

"Yes, she was. Then the king had Claudio brought out of hiding, and Isabella was so happy! Her brother wasn't dead, he was alive! Her brother was alive! Isabella was so, so happy! And Lord Angelo promised to love Jasmine Sarah Savannah and live with her happily. The best part was that the king, who had fallen in love with Isabella, married her and made her the Queen of Vienna!"

"What?" the girls were stunned.

"Isabella became the Queen of Vienna!"

To my surprise, the girls jumped out of bed, pranced, whooped, and clapped.

"Yay! That was a *good* one, Dad! Another! Another!"

CHAPTER 16
BURNED

"Hotspur 9-1-1. What's your emergency?"

"This is Dr. Mathur. I'm at home, 628 High Road, but I just heard someone screaming for help from Memory Lake, down at the bottom of the hill. I can't see what's happening because of the trees and it's dark."

"What kind of emergency, Doc?"

"Not sure. I know someone's badly hurt. I'm going to go and find out."

"You said 628 High Road?"

"Yes."

"Are you in any danger, Doc?"

"No, I'm fine. My family's fine. But there's some serious trouble around Memory Lake. I heard some music and partying earlier, and now there are cries and screams. I can smell smoke."

"Kids often have wild parties down there. Doc, just stay at home, don't go down. I'm sending the sheriff and an ambulance."

"You don't want me to go down?"

"No, Doc. Stay where you are."

"The lake's not far, just at the bottom of the hill. There's a lot of brush and trees, so I can't see the lake itself. Maybe I could help."

The voice paused.

"Doc, there's been some drug deals there. Could get dangerous. Don't go down there. Just stay at home, stay indoors and lock your doors. We'll take it from here."

"Thank you."

"Uh huh."

I hung up and looked at Maya.

"Something's going on. I think there was a party and something went wrong," I said. "There was a lot of music but all that's gone, just loud crying."

"I can smell smoke and barbecue," she said. "And something else, like permed hair."

"I smelled something else, too. Something like barbecue, but different," I said.

"Should we go down there to check?"

"The 911 operator told me to stay at home, because there might be drugs involved."

"Drugs? Here?" Maya was incredulous.

"Yes. It's awful to think that, but yes. There could be a drug deal or just a party with drugs."

Maya stiffened.

"I think we should get a gun. We should have something to defend ourselves, just in case," she said.

I thought about it.

"You know, in India and in England, we never had guns. I'm not very comfortable with the idea of having a gun. Do you really think we need one?"

"How else are you going to protect your own family? What if some druggie came up from Memory Lake and tried to get into our house?" Maya asked, her voice rising.

"I know. That's a scary thought. We do need to be prepared."

"We should be able to defend ourselves. We need a gun!"

"Let me think about it."

"*Think* about it? What's there to think about? Are you going to protect your family or not?"

"Of course I am! But I just haven't ever had a gun. I had an air pistol as a kid, but not a real gun. Let me think about it, just today."

"My vote is to get a gun, a nice gun, that both of us can use. Maybe two, one for me and one for you," Maya said.

I was taken aback.

"*Two* guns?" I said. "Isn't that too much?"

"Agatha and Tommy Templar have two rifles and two guns," Maya said. "This is West Texas, not London. Get real, honey!"

The head nurse at the hospital called fifteen minutes later.

"Doc, the paramedics called us. Some kids from the Air Force were having a party by Memory Lake. They had a fire going and this young pilot threw some gasoline on it. He caught on fire. They got the fire out, but he's burnt pretty bad!"

"That's terrible!"

"Yes. He's in the ER. He needs to be seen ASAP!"

"Dr. Ehrlich is on call, thank goodness."

"We haven't seen him all day. Doc, will you come and see this patient?"

I suppressed my anger and swallowed.

"Will you see the patient?" the nurse asked again.

"I'm not on call!" I exploded.

"I know that," the nurse responded calmly. "But we don't have anyone else and this is a sweet young kid, a pilot, God love him."

"I'm not on call. Get the administrator to call Ehrlich at home and get the hell over here!" I snapped.

The nurse paused.

"Doc, even if I could get Mr. Dawkins to call Dr. Ehrlich at home and even if he agreed to come in, it would take hours. This kid needs help now!"

"This isn't fair," I complained. "Can't you just transfer him to a bigger facility?"

"Simon says he's too critical to transfer. He needs a doctor *right now*," the nurse insisted.

I had no choice. I wondered how I would explain this to Maya and the girls.

"Will you come?" the nurse asked cautiously.

"Yes. Is Simon in the ER?"

"Yes, Doc."

"Tell him to get the history from the friends and family and get ready for a central line."

"Will do, Doc. Thank you."

I explained the situation to Maya. She looked glum.

"I knew Dr. Ehrlich wouldn't come in," Maya said. "He's been mad at you."

The sharp smell of burnt meat struck me in the ER parking lot. There were six trucks parked haphazardly and a purple Lincoln Town Car right next to the ER, underneath the window. I saw that it was occupied, but the doors were shut and the windows closed. About twenty young men and women in jeans and T-shirts shuffled around the doors, voices hushed, faces red with worry. They cringed at the shrieking. I cut through them and swung open the doors of the ER. The corridor was acrid and the screaming grew louder.

A young man lay writhing and howling. Simon and a young woman were trying to lie him down, but he kept getting up.

"No! No!" he yelled and pushed back. "Damn it, damn it, *damn it*, it hurts! My back's burnt!"

Simon saw me and straightened up.

"Thank God you're here!" he said.

The man pushed him back and sat up. He was over six feet, lean, red-haired, and had a crew cut. His hair was burnt and black at the forehead and over the ears. He wore torn jeans and nothing else. His right hand, arm and forearm were swollen, red and blistered like an enormous sausage, and the left hand and forearm had orange postage-stamp sized burns which curled at the corners. His body was covered with fine gray dust and his face was studded with dime-sized swollen blisters. He held his right side stiffly and the slightest movement made him cry out. He turned to show me his back. I walked up to him and was shocked to see that his hair was still smoldering.

"Give me a wet towel!" I ordered.

Simon soaked a towel in tap water and handed it to me. I mopped the man's head. He mumbled, and pointed to his back.

The lower back was crimson and swollen, like charred orange peel, and drops of clear fluid welled up, stuck to each other, and formed brief rivulets. The effort of twisting squeezed more fluid out and he swore. The skin next to the burn hung down in thin white membranes. The man cried again as he untwisted, breathed rapidly, and forced himself to calm down.

"I can't lie down! I can't! I can't! My back's killing me!" he gasped.

Simon handed me the ER chart.

"Dr. Mathur, this is Mr. Brian Vasco. He's a pilot in the U.S. Air Force. He was at a cookout with his friends and attempted to get some sort of bonfire going."

"Barbecue!" Brian rasped. "Barbecue!"

"A barbecue, correct," Simon said.

A young woman stepped forward. She was short and plump, had black hair streaked with purple and small locks hanging from her nose and ears. Her arms and forearms were covered with tattoos.

"He was just trying to get the fire going," the young woman said. "So he opened a can of gasoline and poured it on the fire. I guess the fire jumped up and the can kind of exploded like a hand grenade."

"Who are you?" I asked.

"I'm Sally, Sally Nieves. I'm his fiancée."

I looked at her. I noticed she had short-cut jeans and red boots.

"Is he going to be all right?" she asked nervously.

I scanned the chart. *Brian Rasco, thirty-two, pilot in the US Air Force, based at Lackland Air Force Base in San Antonio, on no medicines, no medical or surgical issues, formerly in excellent health.*

Until this.

"Okay, we're all going to gown up," I ordered. "You too, Miss Nieves. We need to wear gowns and masks and gloves. Brian has serious burns and could get infected."

We slipped into protective gear and I pulled sterile gloves over my regular gloves before examining Brian. His right hand, arm and forearm had nearly doubled in size; they were red and weeping. On his forearms, the skin had curled into rolls of lace. The left side was Anjalilarly affected as well as a patch the size of a shoebox on his back, above the belt line. His face had seven coin-sized burns, on his cheek and neck, and his hair was charred with bald scarlet patches.

"Doc, I need something for pain!" Brian begged.

"Yes, I know. I'm going to give you some morphine. I need to start an IV but your right side is bad. Your left side has multiple burns and your elbow has a second degree burn. I might be able to get one in your left hand. Simon, give me an eighteen gauge butterfly set."

"Go for it, Doc! Just hurry" Brian pleaded.

"He doesn't usually complain, Doctor," Sally said.

I tied a tourniquet just above Brian's wrist.

"I mean it," Sally repeated. "He never complains."

I nodded.

"A month ago he fired a nail into his hand with a nail gun. You know what he did?"

I wiped the back of Brian's hand with alcohol. He winced but said nothing.

"He just pulled it out! Yanked it out!" Sally said.

"Make a fist, Brian!" I ordered.

Brian complied

"Again!" I ordered.

"Pulled the nail out and didn't say a word to me or anyone!" Sally concluded. "Didn't want to ruin my day. He was planning this party."

I inspected the hand.

"Brian, you've got some scarring on your hand. Maybe from the nail gun. You're right handed, so you must have held the nail gun in your right hand and hit the left, correct?"

"Yeah."

"There's a decent vein. I think I can get it. The scar twists it a little."

There was a knock at the door and a lanky young man with red hair appeared.

"Hey Doc! How's my brother?" he asked.

"I'm going to start an IV. It's too soon to tell you anything."

"Mind if I hang around with you here?"

"It's a small room. I don't want to contaminate Brian's burns, so it would be better if you waited outside."

"Sally, Mother wants to come and be with Brian," the young man said.

"That will be too many people," I said.

"She wants you to go, Sally, and then she'll come," Brian's brother continued.

"I'm not leaving Brian," Sally said.

Brian's brother disappeared.

Sally covered her eyes. Simon opened a sterile kit containing an eighteen gauge butterfly catheter.

"Sure you want an eighteen?" Simon asked.

"He's going to need lots of fluids. We need really good access. I could get a smaller one easily, but he needs a wide-bore IV."

"You're taking a chance," Simon cautioned.

I looked at Brian's hand again. The vein had distended after tying the tourniquet. It could easily have handled a smaller catheter, but Brian needed the eighteen.

"Make a fist again!" I ordered. Brian clenched his jaws and squeezed his fist. I slid the sharp metal tip of the catheter into the vein, turning to match the veins contours. I pinned the catheter tip down with my left thumb and pulled the metal stilette out from the hub. Simon whipped off the tourniquet. No blood came out of the catheter.

"You missed it!" Sally cried.

I waited and watched. Nothing.

"You missed it! Hurry up and try again somewhere!" Simon urged.

I withdrew the catheter a fraction.

"It's not working, Doctor! It's not working!" Sally shrieked.

I pulled the catheter out a little more. A bead of blood appeared at the end of the catheter.

"Hey! How about that! You're in after all!" Simon whooped. "Here, let me connect the IV."

"Sometimes you're up against a valve in the vein, so you just have to withdraw a little," I explained.

I twisted the plastic catheter a little and advanced it again. It continued to drip blood.

"Ringer's lactate, wide open. Give him a thousand cc stat. Then three hundred an hour. You got the morphine?"

"Ready!"

"Four of morphine now, give twenty five of Phenergan as well."

I taped the catheter down securely. I taped the plastic tubing to his middle finger for further security.

"No burns below your waist?"

"No."

"No burns in your private parts, your backside or your thighs or legs?"

"No."

"Okay, let's wash the burns with saline and apply silver sulfadiazine. We're going to need a lot, Simon!"

"Very good, Dr. Mathur! I'll be right back from the pharmacy. Here's your sterile saline," Simon said.

"I asked for Ringer's lactate!" I exclaimed.

"Terribly sorry, Doctor! We're all out of Ringer's. But we do have an awful lot of saline!"

"Why are we out of Ringer's lactate?"

"Because vendors like to get paid. They won't give us any RL if we don't pay for it," Simon explained. "Understandable, wouldn't you say?"

"I understand. But I thought the hospital was doing well now, financially."

"It was. It is. But we've had all these old bills from our vendors for three years and it's going to take several more years to pay them off."

I connected the bag of saline to the IV tubing.

"Call San Antonio. Tell them we need to transfer him there ASAP. We can send him in an ambulance or helicopter."

Simon turned to Brian.

"I need your driver's license and your social security number, and your Air Force ID," he said. Sally emptied a plastic bag. A wallet, a key chain and a pair of thick glasses fell out. She opened his wallet and extracted two cards.

"His social is on the Air Force ID," she said.

I stared at the glasses.

"Pretty thick glasses for a pilot," Simon said.

"Those are mine," Sally said, hastily.

"Lucky your eyes were spared," I said to Brian.

"Uh huh," he nodded, without emotion.

He started to relax after getting the morphine. I lifted up the back of the gurney and he tried to rest on it but couldn't.

"My back really hurts," Brian complained. "I can't put any pressure on it."

"Okay, stay sitting for now. I'm going to start cleaning your right side, then your face," I said.

I placed fresh towels around his neck and squirted sterile saline on the damaged areas of his right arm and forearm. Brian winced and withdrew, then steadied himself.

"You've got burns on your forehead and your cheeks but not on your eyelids. No pain in your eyes? Does it hurt to move your eyes from side to side?"

Brian rolled his eyeballs cautiously.

"Nope," he answered.

"Good. Then there's no corneal damage. The cornea is the clear part of the eye. If there was any damage there, it would be very painful."

"No pain there," Brian mumbled.

"He's getting sleepy," Sally observed.

"I'm going to look at your back, Brian. Sit up straight, please." Brian shook his head wearily and straightened up. Simon whistled.

"By Jove! That's a bugger!" he exclaimed.

"What?" Brian jerked up, wide awake.

"You've got a large blister on one corner of the burn, it's about two inches wide, over your back. It may burst when I clean it," I said.

I placed towels behind him and tied one around his waist.

"I don't want to wet your trousers," I explained.

Brian's head drooped again. He said nothing. Sally and Simon watched him warily.

"I'm starting now," I warned.

I washed the burn carefully.

"It's a large one," I went on, "about twelve inches by eight inches, looks angry."

Brian swayed a little.

"But there is a silver lining," I murmured.

I sprayed the blister with saline. Brian jerked again.

"How can there be a silver lining to this?" Sally asked.

I took a piece of gauze, soaked it in iodine, and wiped the blister. It remained intact. Encouraged, I washed and wiped again. The blister ruptured and the pale membrane peeled off. Before I could pull back, I touched the skin next to the burn with the gauze. Brian screamed and twisted. He lunged at me with his left hand. The pole and bag of saline crashed to the floor and Brian kept screaming.

"Good Lord!" Simon shrieked. "Look at the bloody IV!"

The IV cannula had pulled out and had ripped off a ribbon of burned red flesh six inches long and an inch wide. It fluttered like a pendant. Brian waved his hand in horror, trying to shake it loose. Drops of blood popped out and splattered the floor.

Brian screamed again and his brother's head re-appeared.

"I have to cut off the IV! Get me some gauze and a fifteen blade!" I ordered.

"Help me!" Brian screamed. "Help! Help!"

Sally cried and rushed to his side and wavered helplessly.

His brother stepped in.

"Get out!" I yelled.

The brother looked confused.

"Do something for him!" Sally begged. "Look at his hand! He's ripped the whole skin off!"

"Simon! Put on sterile gloves! I need a fifteen blade. Hold him!"

Simon broke out of his shock and rushed into action.

"Hold him!" I repeated.

Simon held him at the wrist and elbow.

"Steady! I'm going to cut the IV out of the skin."

I held the skin flap down with the gauze and dissected the IV cannula off. I washed both sides of the skin flap and gently replaced it on its bed. Brian watched it all, shaking.

"You want to tape it down?" Simon asked.

"Yes, with paper tape. Not regular tape."

"I'll get it from the nurses station." Simon peeled off his gloves and ran.

Brian was racked with pain. I picked up a syringe and drew up morphine. His brother cleared his throat and spoke.

"Mother wants to come in and be with Brian," the brother repeated, forcefully.

Sally glared at him.

"Tell her she can come," she said.

"Mother wants you to leave," the brother said. "She doesn't want to be in here with you. She wants to be here with Brian."

"I'm not leaving," Sally insisted.

Brian coughed and spoke up.

"Tell Mother I've always done whatever she wanted, always. Now this one time in my life I want to do something, she won't let me!"

"Mother wants to be with you, Brian."

"Tell her she has to accept Sally first," Brian said. "I want to get engaged to Sally and marry her."

Brian's brother shook his head and left.

"Tell Mother I love her," Brian called out. "Tell her! Tell her, I've always done everything she wanted! Can't she do this for me?"

There was an awkward silence.

"What's the silver lining?" Sally asked.

"What?"

"You were saying something about a silver lining," she reminded me.

I removed Brian's shoes and socks and rolled up his jeans. I scanned his feet for suitable veins.

"We may have to start an IV here," I said.

"What was the silver lining?" Sally repeated.

"The silver lining is that Brian is feeling a lot of pain. That means that the nerves are still working. In really bad burns, third degree burns, there's no pain because the nerves are burnt and not working. So the pain means that Brian's nerves are still working, they didn't get destroyed."

Brian controlled his breathing.

"So pain is good," Brian whispered.

"In this case, yes," I answered.

Sally peered over my shoulder.

"Do you see a good vein in his foot?" she asked.

"No, his veins here are too small. I could start a small butterfly needle IV but that wouldn't help much," I said.

I tied tourniquets above his ankles and moved his feet, and looked from different angles.

"What if you don't find a good vein in the foot or the leg?" Sally asked.

"I could start one in the groin," I said. Brian winced and

shook his head.

"But there's a risk of infection," I continued. "The groin is warm and moist and full of bacteria. So I don't like starting IVs there."

"Then where else?" Sally persisted.

"I may have to put one in his neck."

"His neck!" Sally was alarmed. "Isn't that really risky? Sticking him in the neck?"

I hesitated.

"Well, yes. There's some risk. The vein lies just to the side of the artery. So if I miss and hit the artery instead of the vein, that would be bad."

"How bad? What does that artery do?" Sally asked.

"It carries blood to the brain."

"So Brian could have brain damage?" Sally cried, horrified.

"It's possible. But rare."

"Have you done many neck IVs?"

"Over a hundred."

"Any complications?"

"None so far."

Sally exhaled slowly. Simon bounded in with the paper tape.

"Got it! You want to give some morphine first?" he asked.

"Yes. You need to chart it and draw it up. I need to sign for it and the previous dose."

Simon scribbled and handed me the chart. He taped down the torn flap of skin with the paper tape.

"You can give him back his driver's license; it's under the clip."

I glanced at the license, then held it in front of him.

"There's something wrong," I said.

Brian peered at it.

"What's wrong?" he asked.

"Expired," I said, "six months ago."

Sally snatched it and looked.

"Crud! He's right!"

"Strange that he couldn't read it, but you could," I said.

"Why?"

"*You're* the one with glasses, Sally. But you read it without glasses."

Sally was flustered.

"Those are for distance," she explained.

I picked up the glasses and held them just above the chart. I moved the glasses backwards and forwards.

"The words keep changing. Sometimes they are inverted and sometimes upright, and their size varies as well. Those are convex lenses. These glasses are for people who can't see close up," I said, quietly. "And you can see close up, Sally."

Brian and Sally looked at each other.

"You're right," Brian admitted. "Those are my glasses."

"Brian's having some eye problems. He can't see up close. We're trying to get him in with a specialist in Austin. If his eyesight gets bad, he won't be able to fly," Sally said.

"I have an appointment to see the specialist next week. I was hoping to see him without making a big deal about it. I don't want to lose my wings," Brian added.

"Brian, when you picked up the gasoline, did you pick it up by mistake?" I asked.

Brian gave a hollow laugh.

"Yes. Wasn't wearing my glasses, grabbed the wrong bottle. Couldn't read the damn label, thought it was water."

"What a screw-up!" Sally said. "Just when we thought we had it all planned and figured out!"

Simon handed me the morphine vial and the loaded

syringe. I checked the contents and the expiry date.

"The best laid plans of mice and men sometimes go awry," he said.

I nodded.

"Please read and sign the consent for the jugular IV line before I give you any more morphine," I told Brian.

Sally slipped the glasses on Brian and he scanned the document, nodded and initialed it. I injected morphine into his deltoid muscle. A few minutes later, Brian sighed and slumped again.

"Why didn't you give it IV?" Simon asked.

"I chose to give the morphine intramuscularly, not IV. Shots into the muscle take a little longer to start but last longer," I explained.

"I just wanted to have a family. I wanted to keep my job. I love flying," Brian said, sleepily.

"Just relax, baby," Sally said, holding his ankle. "Relax. Let the medicine work."

"I know I did wrong by hiding my eye problems, but I wanted to keep flying and get married and have kids and all, you know," Brian said.

"Your voice is slurring," Simon said. "Looks like the morphine is hitting you."

"I feel it, feels good, good," Brian mumbled.

"We need to lie him down," I instructed Simon. "Then get ready for a right internal jugular central line. He has no IV access right now."

"How about a femoral line in the groin? Dr. Becker puts in femoral lines," Simon said.

"I'm aware of that. But the groin is a dirty place. I don't want him to get an infection."

"A femoral line is much easier!"

"I know that. A jugular line is cleaner and safer."

"But you could hit the carotid artery in the neck," Simon persisted.

I nodded, hoping Simon would stop.

"He could hemorrhage! He could bleed out!" Simon hissed.

"I know."

"Stroke! He could have a stroke!" Simon whispered.

I glared at Simon.

"Simon, I'm aware of the risks. Let's get the set open, get him down slowly and drape the chest and head and left side of the neck."

"He's so young," Simon continued, quietly. "Hate for him to have a stroke or bleed to death. What with your luck recently."

Sally was close to tears. I glared at Simon.

"Brian looks sleepy," I said, and eased him down.

Sally had been listening.

"Could he die if you mess up?" Sally whispered.

"Highly unlikely," I replied.

"You mean, it's possible?" she persisted.

"Look, all the things Simon said are true, it's *possible* that Brian could have massive bleeding or a stroke. But it's not *probable*."

"Please be careful!" Sally pleaded.

I nodded. Sally hesitated.

"We plan to get engaged this summer. We were going to announce it to our friends today. That's what the party was about."

"What about his eye problems?" I asked.

"We were going to see a specialist in Austin, and if there was no hope, then Brian would resign from the Air Force and move back to Hotspur."

"Are you from Hotspur?" Simon asked.

"No, but Brian is. His parents have land. The Hawthorne ranch. His mother's a Hawthorne."

Simon gave a low whistle.

"That's the big ranch that has oil wells and windmills," he said.

Brian was drowsy. I placed a towel under his head and slipped on fresh sterile gloves. I painted his neck with iodine and wiped it off with alcohol. The smell of iodine and alcohol reminded me of my days as a junior doctor in London. I had placed so many jugular lines there that I felt confident.

Simon trained the overhead light on the right side of the neck. I draped everything else, leaving only a rectangle of skin visible.

I placed the fingertips of my left hand on the right carotid artery in the neck. With my right hand, I grasped a ten cc syringe, filled it with lidocaine, and snapped on a twenty-two gauge inch-long needle. Sally moved away and covered her eyes.

"Maybe that wasn't sensible to hide Brian's bad eyesight," she said.

I inserted the needle at a forty-five degree angle, just to the side of my middle left finger. As I advanced the needle, I pulled back on the plunger, creating suction. I advanced the needle cautiously. Nothing happened. I withdrew and started again, a little more to the side. Nothing. No blood return.

The door swung open and Brian's brother returned.

"Hey, Doc, how's he doing?" he asked.

Sally ignored him. She gazed at me fixedly, avoiding a downward look at Brian's neck.

"It's not working?" Sally asked me, nervously.

"No," I admitted.

"What's not working?" his brother echoed.

"You said you've done this before," Sally said, her voice

rising.

"What's the problem?" his brother repeated, his tone rising. I ignored him too.

"Yes, Sally, I have done this many times. Many times. Be patient."

"What's the damn problem, for God's sake?" his brother demanded.

"He's dehydrated. His veins are flat. Let's lower the head end of the bed. That should fill up his jugular veins."

Simon lowered the head end. Sally started pacing the floor. The brother advanced into the room cautiously and stood behind me.

"What do we do if you still don't get in?" he asked.

"You need to step out. I told you, this is a small room and I don't want you in here."

He withdrew but stood stubbornly by the door and crossed his arms.

"What are you going to do if you don't get in?" he asked again.

"Then I'll start a femoral line. In his groin."

"But you said that would give him an infection!" Sally said.

"We've got to get him IV access! Be quiet! Let me focus," I growled.

I waited a moment, then inserted the needle a third time, same angle, but a little closer to the jaw. I pulled back on the plunger and advanced.

Nothing.

"Dang! Dang it! Do something!" Sally wailed.

I withdrew the needle slowly. As I came out, a thread of crimson fluid curled into the syringe.

"You're in!" Simon cried. "Great job! You got it!"

I glanced at Sally. She was trembling.

"Oh, thank God, thank God, thank God!" she whispered. She clasped her hands and looked up.

"It's not over yet. Give me the big needle," I said.

Simon pulled on sterile gloves and located the metal needle in the pack.

"That's a freaking big needle!" Sally cried out.

"Yes, it is. I used the thin needle to find the vein, now I'm going to get into it with the big needle."

"Why didn't you start with the big needle?"

"I didn't want to poke around his neck with a big needle. I use the thin needle to find the vein, then the big needle to get into it."

"That's a jolly big needle!" Simon declared. Sally shuddered. Brian's brother jumped out into the corridor.

"Better look away," I advised.

Sally walked to the window and looked out at the purple Lincoln parked right next to the ER.

"His mother is in the car," she observed. "She won't come in."

"Why not?" Simon asked.

"She doesn't like me. I'm divorced. I have a daughter. They don't approve of me."

"I see."

"And I'm from Massachusetts. I'm a Yankee, don't hunt or shoot, talk too much. She says I'm a Masshole. We're always fighting."

"You don't hunt or shoot? Do you know how to fire a gun?" Simon asked.

"No. I don't like guns," Sally said. "Another black mark."

"In Texas, everyone has a gun. You really have to have a gun. Right, Doctor?" Simon said.

I shrugged.

"The latest fight was because I wouldn't let Brian go hunting with them," Sally continued. "Hunting! No sense in it. I say it's just not worth it. No sense in hunting, I think, not worth the risk."

"Then let us pray that come it may," Simon recited. "That sense and worth, over all the earth, shall bear the gree and that."

I was surprised.

"The gree? What in the world are you saying?" I said.

"A spot of poetry seemed appropriate," Simon winked.

I returned to Brian's neck and wiped away a trickle of blood from the puncture site. I was irritated. I didn't understand what Simon had said. I decided to focus and carry on.

"Simon, pay attention! I'm going in with the big needle. I'm going to need the guide wire," I snapped.

Simon sprung to attention.

I peered at Brian's neck. I had to retrace the path of the thinner needle with the large needle. I thrust the large needle on top of a twenty cc syringe, then punctured the neck with the big needle, and advanced millimeter by millimeter in the same direction. Brian didn't budge, and I marvelled at the numbing effect of lidocaine. There was a gratifying surge of blood.

"Give me the guide wire!" I commanded.

I threaded the guide wire through the metal needle. I withdrew the needle, leaving the guide wire in the vein. I pressed down on the neck with gauze to stop the flow of blood.

"Now give me the big plastic cannula."

Simon handed me a white tube, as thick as a shoelace. I slid it over the free end of the guidewire and into the neck until only an inch was left outside. There were two perforated flaps. I removed the guide wire, leaving the plastic cannula in the external jugular vein.

"There's a burnt area nearby. I have to stitch the flaps to the skin so the catheter doesn't come out."

"Be careful! We don't want the burnt skin to peel off like it did on his hand!" Sally warned.

I nodded. As I stitched the cannula in place, I thought back.

"What were you saying earlier, Simon?" I asked.

"Poetry. I was reciting poetry."

"Poetry? Now?"

"Like I said, it seemed appropriate."

I glanced at him, still puzzled. He grinned infuriatingly but gave no clue. I decided to forget about it. It was diverting my attention.

"I need to call San Antonio. I'm going to stitch this cannula in and then tape it down with some Tegaderm. Keep another four milligrams of morphine ready," I said.

"Right you are, Doctor!"

"Let's give him five hundred of saline wide open for one bag then three hundred cc per hour."

"Getting it right now!"

"We need to apply silver sulfadiazine ointment on the burnt areas, now that I've washed them," I said, and showed Simon how to apply the ointment gently and evenly. Sally came back and watched, and grasped Brian's bare feet. Brian moaned and struggled to wake up. His brother stepped in again. I was too weary to object and let him hover by the door.

"Are you hurting, love?" Sally asked. Brian nodded.

"Give two more milligrams of morphine IV," I ordered. "Two, not four."

Simon injected the morphine.

"You've had eight milligrams of morphine so far, sir. Now you're getting another two. Ten milligrams in all," I said.

"Is that a lot?" Sally asked.

"That's what I give for a heart attack," I said.

"He's been hurt badly, madam. He needed it," Simon reassured her.

Sally nodded. She rubbed Brian's feet slowly.

"I love you, Brian," she whispered.

Brian stirred and shook his head.

"Love? Me? All burned up? Ugly, blind, unemployed?" Brian asked.

"You don't know how much I love you," Sally said, her voice quivering.

I stepped into the dictation room and sat down with the paperwork. I called the Emergency Center at Lackland Air Force Base. I was connected to Major Sheldon.

"I've been expecting your call. Brian's buddies called me, told me what happened. How bad is it?" he asked, bluntly.

"Pretty bad. Second degree burns all of the right upper limb, right side of face, part of the scalp, patches on the left upper limb and a six by nine inch area on the lower back."

"So what percentage?"

"About twenty to thirty percent of the body."

There was a pause.

"That's bad," Major Sheldon muttered.

"But he's young and healthy. He can make it."

"Yeah, maybe. Career's screwed. Eyes okay?"

I hesitated.

"Not burned," I said, truthfully.

"Huh. Maybe there's hope. Did you get in the lines?"

"I put in one central line, right jugular."

"He needs two lines. Stitch them in. Do it before you ship him," Major Sheldon ordered.

"I can do a foot IV or a femoral," I offered.

"Foot veins can be tricky. Don't want a blood clot."

"Then I can do a femoral line," I said, without enthusiasm.

Major Sheldon thought for a moment.

"No. Go with the foot. Those femoral lines in the groin tend to get infected."

"Will do. We have the ambulance ready and we can have him out of here in fifteen minutes" I said.

"Good! Remember, stitch both the IVs to the skin! We have to have good venous access. Plenty of fluids!"

I thanked him and hung up. I walked back to the main room. Simon was talking to Sally.

"We need to start another IV in his foot," I announced.

"Would you like me to try?" Simon asked.

"No, it's difficult. Let me go ahead. Let's clean up the right foot and put a tourniquet on the ankle."

Simon rolled up Brian's jeans.

"Should we just take off the jeans?" he wondered.

"No, leave them on. He's at risk of hypothermia."

"What's that?" Sally asked.

"He's at risk of losing body heat," I explained. "The loss of skin covering means he has no insulation in many areas. So his body could cool down too much. I've covered the burns with ointment but that's not as good as healthy skin. Let's conserve whatever heat we can."

Simon cleaned the right foot with soapy water, then with iodine. I fastened a tourniquet at the ankle and put on gloves. A foot vein stood out above the instep. I was able to get a thin catheter into it. Brian woke up with the stab.

"Damn it! Damn it, that hurts!" he moaned.

I stood up and peeled off my gloves and hurled them into the bin.

"Done! I'm finally done! Simon, please stitch that IV in place. I've written my notes, so make photocopies and send them with Brian. I'm going home."

I ripped off my cap, face mask and gown and retreated into the corridor. Simon silently handed me another ER chart.

"What?" I burst out. "*What?* Are you *kidding* me?"

"Before you got here, another patient showed up. His name's Dell Clawsom. He says he has a chest infection and just wants a shot," he said. I refused the chart and shook my head.

"No! No! You didn't tell me about him," I complained. "It's almost ten. I need to go home."

"I told him you weren't on call. When I said you were coming in, he said he would wait for you at the nurses' station."

"Is he still here?"

"Yes. I just saw him when I went to get the paper tape."

I stared at Simon in shock and anger.

"Sorry. Not kidding," Simon shrugged. "But Mr. Clawsom is pretty well-known around here. Maybe he could write you a letter for your green card interview?"

After the debacle with Mr. Rutherford, I needed someone in my corner. Maybe this would help the family, I thought. I wavered.

"Put him in room two," I sighed.

"I already did."

"Is he upset because he had to wait so long?"

"No, he's very understanding."

"Did you read him some poetry? To calm the savage beast? Sing a few songs?"

"I detect some sarcasm, Doctor."

"You detect accurately."

"You object to my recitation?" Simon asked, drily.

"I know you're doing it for a reason. I just can't figure out why."

Simon smiled.

"Then you won't mind if I give the young lady a poem to recite to her fiancé?"

"A poem? What is wrong with you?" I said. "This is ridiculous!"

"I already asked her while you were talking to San Antonio. She says she would like to read it out to him."

"Simon, what is the purpose of all this?"

"Because she loves Brian."

I waved the ER chart in surrender.

"I'm going to Room Two, and I want to get done as soon as possible. Read the poem yourself or she can read it, that's fine, I don't care, just get him ready for the ambulance," I said.

"Thank you, Doctor," Simon bowed with exaggerated courtesy.

I stepped into the corridor and reviewed the chart. Dell Clawsom was a seventy-one year old man who lived in Tuscola, a tiny community about thirty miles west of Hotspur. He was on captopril and Lasix and was allergic to iodine. He had multiple abdominal and back surgeries. His main problem was shortness of breath for a week. Before I could enter Room Two, I heard Sally and froze.

"My love is like a red, red rose
That's newly sprung in June,
Oh, my heart is like the melody
That's sweetly sung in tune."

I remembered the verse and it finally made sense. I groaned. Simon was celebrating Burns night.

CHAPTER 17

AWESOME DELL CLAWSOM

The door in front of me swung open and I saw a tall, thin man with a mop of sticky white hair. He wore stringy denim overalls over a tattered T-shirt. He emanated turpentine.

"Dell Clawsom!" he said enthusiastically. "Good to meet you!"

"Thanks for waiting. I'm Dr. Mathur."

"I figured. The white coat and stethoscope are a dead giveaway, Doc!" he laughed.

I stepped into Room Two. It was half the size of the other room, square, windowless, and lit up with six fluorescent tube lights. There was a metal ladder in the corner and dust all over the floor, stools, and examination table. I remembered they had just repaired the roof.

"I know you're busy," he said. "I just need a shot. I'll be good to go! I'll get out of here and you can go home too."

"Hang on. I know you're in a hurry. Just sit down for a minute."

Dell dusted the edge of the chair and sat down.

"Just give me a shot, Doc. That's all I need! I know my body!" he insisted.

"What's the problem, exactly?"

Dell shook his head and looked at the ceiling.

"Pneumonia," he stated, as if stating the obvious.

"You're short of breath?"

"Bingo!"

"For a week?"

"Yup."

"Any cough?"
"Nope."
"Wheezing?"
"Nope."
"Heart problems?"
"Never."
"Any other medical problems, besides high blood pressure?"

Dell looked up.

"How'd you know?"

"You're on captopril and Lasix. It's on the chart."

"Oh, yeah. But I'm in great health, Doc! I'm a pilot, see? I get physicals every year so that I can fly. Just had one, did every test known to man and then some!"

"You look pale. Were your labs normal?"

"Perfect!"

"Let me examine you."

Dell shrugged. He slipped down his overall straps and pulled up his vest.

"Go right ahead!"

I examined him swiftly, then straightened up.

"Your heart rate is fast, your eyes are pale, but your lungs are clear."

Dell looked at me in surprise.

"Clear?"

"Totally clear. I think you're anemic, or low in blood. That's why you're short of breath."

Dell shook his head in disbelief.

"I just had my flight physical six months ago, Doc. Labs, stress test, the works! Stone cold normal. Just pneumonia, that's all. I guarantee it."

I shook my head wearily.

"Mr. Clawsom," I began.

He immediately held up his hand.

"Dell. Call me Dell."

"Dell, I'm tired and don't want to argue. Let's do both. Let's get a blood count to check for anemia and a chest X-ray for pneumonia."

"How long Is that going to take?"

"An hour."

Dell groaned.

"Just give me the shot, Doc! I'll get out of your hair!"

I hesitated.

"Doc, go home to your wife and kiddos! They must be missing you. You spend all this time in the hospital, you really need to be home."

I looked at him again. He was very pale.

"No. No shot until we do the tests," I insisted.

Dell slumped.

"You're killing me, Doc! Just give me the shot! I want to go home, you want to go home too, right?" he pleaded.

I write my note in silence. I was dying to go home.

"Do the tests first," I ordered.

"It's going to take forever!" he grumbled.

I went back to Room One and handed Simon the chart. He glanced at it.

"You want a CBC and a chest X-ray? That's going to take some time!"

"I know. Call me at home with the results," I said.

"Mr. Clawsom agreed?" Simon asked.

"He didn't say no," I replied. Simon shook his head

"He won't agree," Simon said.

"His lungs are clear, and he looks pale. He thinks he has pneumonia and wants a shot. I don't see the evidence for pneumonia."

"How about a compromise? Give him the shot now, and do the labs tomorrow?"

I hesitated.

"It's late," Simon observed, "and you're tired. Be easy on yourself, Doctor."

"Here's the compromise. Do the labs now, and come back in the morning for the shot, *after* I see the X ray and the blood tests."

"You're a hard man!" Simon complained.

"That's what the actress said to the bishop, right?" I retorted.

Simon grinned and left to arrange the tests.

The paramedics had moved Brian to their mobile stretcher and strapped him in securely. Brian was sleepy; his head kept dropping. Sally went over the paperwork and collected Brian's belongings. I examined Brian's skin and the IV sites. I listened to his heart and lungs again.

"What if he starts hurting again before we get there?" Sally asked.

"He can have another four milligrams of morphine."

"What if they give him too much?"

"We have a great antidote called Narcan. It reverses morphine completely."

Simon returned and gave a thumbs up. He gathered the paperwork, checked it, and went over it with the paramedics. Sally hugged us awkwardly.

"Thank you both," she said. "You were, ah, awesome!"

"All the best to you and Brian," I said. "You have a long road ahead."

"Literally," Simon added. "Over two hundred miles."

"This evening is going to change our lives forever, I realize that," Sally said. She waved as she accompanied Brian out the room.

"What about Mr. Clawsom in Room Two?" I asked Brian.

"He went to the lab for the tests. He wasn't happy."

"It's already one in the morning. He can get his shot in eight or nine hours."

"Why are you being so contrary? Why won't you just give him a shot?" Simon complained.

"Because he doesn't need it. Again, unnecessary antibiotics. It's the wrong thing to do, so I won't give him the shot," I insisted, gritting my teeth. I was exhausted, snappish, and reckless.

"He won't like you."

"I guess not," I answered, glumly.

"Some rise by sin, and some by virtue fall," Simon sighed.

"You've said that before. *Measure For Measure*."

"Mr. Clawsom wasn't happy. I suspect he won't be writing a letter of support for your green card."

"I don't care. I'm really tired, and I'm going home. Don't call me unless someone is vomiting blood or dying."

The phone rang at seven in the morning.

"*What?*" I snarled.

"Good morning, Dr. Mathur. This is Simon in the Emergency Room."

I took a breath and forced myself to be calm.

"Good morning, Simon," I replied, matching his tone. "Is someone dead or dying?"

"Not at this moment, sir. Do you remember Mr. Clawsom from last night?"

"Of course I do."

"Well, he's back. He got the message you left for him and he's not very happy."

I stifled an urge to scream.

"I waited in the hospital to read his chest X-ray. He was on his way home so I called and left a message on his home phone that it was clear. No pneumonia. But his hemoglobin was eight-point-two. Normal is twelve to fourteen."

"So he is anemic," Simon agreed.

"Absolutely. They called me at three in the morning because it was a critical level."

Simon was not impressed. No sympathetic warbling followed.

"At three in the morning!" I repeated, indignantly.

"Naturally, because it was critical," Simon repeated, calmly. "May I ask what you advised?"

"I had them get two units of blood ready for transfusion."

"The blood is here. But the blood bank in Abilene flagged it."

"Why?"

"Mr. Clawsom has several antibodies in his blood and he may have a reaction to the transfusion. He may have a transfusion reaction."

I sat up in bed, alarmed.

"That could be serious. Where is he?"

"He's with me here in the Emergency Room. I'm looking at him."

"Is he having any chest pain or shortness of breath?"

"No."

"Send him to the Admissions Office and make a fresh ER chart on him. I'll come down for the blood transfusion. Do not start the blood till I get there, he could have a life-threatening reaction. Start a wide-bore IV, preferably an eighteen gauge, and give him fifty milligrams of Benadryl IV now. But don't start the blood until I get there!"

"What about your clinic?"

"I just have one patient this morning. I've already had two

cancellations. What about the crash cart? Has it been restocked?"

"I checked the crash cart and the medications. Everything's there."

"Epinephrine? Lidocaine? Solu-Medrol?"

"Everything's restocked."

"Good. Let's hope we don't need it."

Dell Clawsom was examining the IV in his elbow when I arrived. He was still in threadbare overalls with the ragged T-shirt and reeked of turpentine.

"Don't bend your elbow, sir!" Simon warned.

Dell looked up.

"You have terrible veins, sir! It took me a long time to find that one. If you bend your elbow, you'll kink the IV and it might clot off."

Dell shrugged.

"Absolute disaster!" Simon continued.

"Still smells of burnt hair in here," Dell said.

"Yes, we had a patient here last night," Simon said. "Wretched soul."

"I know, I was here," Dell said. "I heard a lot of crying. I heard some singing, too."

"That was poetry," Simon nodded. "Did you hear the words of the poem?"

"Red roses?" Dell guessed.

"Close enough. Actually, it was, *My love is like a red, red rose.*"

"Robert Burns?"

"Exactly. Very good!" Simon beamed.

Dell nodded.

"Because you had a patient with burns?" Dell asked, smiling.

"That made it Burns Night," Simon nodded. "Only Dr.

Mathur didn't get it. Completely ruined it!"

"I did get it, only later that night," I protested.

Simon shook his head.

"This is the British Hospital of Texas. The Dallas paper said so," Simon explained. "So we had to have a Burns night. And we did."

"Did you give Mr. Clawsom the Benadryl?" I asked.

"Yes, Doctor."

"Let's give twenty of Solu-Medrol as well."

"What's that?" Dell asked.

"That's a steroid. To help prevent an allergic reaction during the blood transfusion. Just being cautious."

Dell reached over and squeezed my arm.

"Relax, Doc. Nothing's going to happen to me. I guarantee it," Dell insisted.

"How do you know that?" I asked, and sat down on a stool next to him.

"Doc, I've been all over the world. Lived in Africa and South America. Bitten and stung by every kind of bug there is, so my blood has all these crazy antibodies."

"The blood bank was concerned, so they alerted us. People can die of a transfusion reaction."

"I'm not going to die of a reaction to blood!"

"I hope not. But I'm not taking any chances. You never know."

Dell shook his head.

"I've been close to death so many times I kind of know. I could have died in Biafra, or in Venezuela, or in Costa Rica. But not in my hometown of Hotspur. I don't think so," he said.

"You mean, you just feel confident."

"No. I *know*. I know I'm not going to have a reaction today. I just know it."

"Okay, let's say that you're right. But I will stay here, at least for the first thirty minutes or so."

"Don't you have patients to see, Doc?" Dell inquired, smirking.

"Not right now."

"How come, Doc?" Dell persisted.

"Because I had two cancellations."

"Why did they cancel?"

"They had to go to the beauty shop."

Dell laughed and slapped his thigh.

"Beauty shop! The doctor got dumped for the beauty shop!" he said, with mock disbelief.

"Yes. They wanted to go to the beauty shop. Didn't care about their blood pressure or heart disease or diabetes, had to get their hair done first," I said, bitterly.

"Hey, don't get upset. That's important in small towns!"

Simon flattened the gurney. Dell tossed him the pillow and lowered his frame gingerly. Simon inserted the pillow under his neck and Dell settled down.

"I have arthritis in my neck," Dell explained, "but if I can get this danged pillow just right, I'll be okay."

Simon flushed the line with sterile saline and started the blood.

"Do you take ibuprofen or something else for neck pain?" I asked.

"Sure do. Every day. Why?"

"Because those medicines can cause stomach bleeding, that might be why you're anemic."

"I had a normal stomach exam and colon exam a year ago."

"Why did you have them done?"

"Flight physical. I'm a pilot."

"You fly for the airlines?"

"No. I fly my own planes."

"You have planes?"

Dell looked at me in mock anger.

"I don't look like I could have planes?"

I shrugged.

"I got a bunch of planes," Dell said. "I restore them."

I listened to Dell's heart and lungs and palpated his abdomen. Everything was normal.

I sat down and started writing notes. Dell looked around and caught Simon's eye.

"Why was this called a British Hospital?" he asked.

"Well, Dr. Mathur trained in London, and I grew up just outside London, near Heathrow Airport. We have several patients who are from England, like my aunt, Mrs. Doris Marsh, and Mrs. Gladys Flynn. We had a reporter from Dallas one evening and she came up with the name," Simon explained.

Dell nodded. I watched him breathe.

"Any difficulty breathing?" I asked.

"No."

"Any chest pain?"

"No."

"Any itching?"

"No."

"Good," I said. "If you feel bad, tell me right away."

Dell grunted. Simon sat down on the other stool. There was silence for a few minutes.

"British Hospital, eh? I got a British story for you," Dell announced.

"Okay," I grunted. I pulled up a stool and sat down in front of the heart monitor.

"In the sixties, I used to work for an oil company called GeoSurvey. We had an interest in Uganda and I sent one of our best engineers, a guy called Stuart Fletcher, to Kinshasa, the capital of Uganda. The big guy in Uganda was this crazy general called Dada Idi Amin. Well, we made him a deal to survey Uganda for oil, and he signed on. Then he changed his mind."

"Why?"

"Money. He wanted more money. So we made another deal. That was a mistake."

"A mistake?"

"He got greedy. Wanted even more. So we canceled everything and I ordered Fletch to come home. You know what Idi Amin did? He put poor Fletch under house arrest."

"So he held Fletcher for ransom, basically?"

"Yep. State-sponsored kidnapping. Couple armed guards with him all the time. Took away his passport, froze his bank account, the works."

"So what did you do?"

"At that time, I was in Kenya, which is next door to Uganda. I'm pretty good with planes, so I figured a plan. There was a big flat park an hour outside of Kinshasa. I got word to Fletch to be there Sunday morning when it's deserted on account of church, just say that he's going for a picnic, give the guards some booze, and slip away. Figured I'd land my little Cessna there and grab him and fly him the heck out of there."

Dell looked at the blood dripping out of the bag into the IV tubing.

"It's fine," Simon assured him.

"Go on," I said.

"So the next Sunday afternoon I get into my Cessna 206, and I fly into Uganda. But there was a mountain range there and a whole lot of fog. Fog so thick you could cut it with a knife! I flew right into the fog and couldn't see a thing. I was scared to death I was going to crash into the mountains!"

"What about radar and navigation?"

"Didn't have it. Just eyes and radio. So I climbed up as high as I could, and called out on the radio for help, and prayed that the Uganda air force didn't hear me first."

"You just called out on the radio for help?"

"I just called around on different frequencies, and asked if the fog had cleared up ahead, and at what altitude."

"What happened?"

"A British guy answered. He told me there was no fog at eight hundred feet. Gave me the coordinates. So I prayed some more and came down through the fog. You know what?"

"What?"

"He was wrong! There was fog at eight hundred feet so I came down some more. Six hundred feet, still fog! Five hundred feet, still fog! What the heck should I do? Couldn't see a darn thing. Reckon I pissed in my pants."

"So what did you do?"

"I prayed. Then I dropped some more. At four hundred feet, it was clear!"

"Then you could see the landmarks?"

"Didn't know any landmarks. I had used up all my gas. There was no way I could reach the park in Uganda and bring Fletch. So I turned back. Didn't even have the gas to make it to Nairobi."

"Did you just land on a field in Kenya?"

"No. I got back on the radio. British guy guided me to an airstrip I never knew about. I landed there to refuel."

"Not in Nairobi?"

"Heck no! I was way low on gas! I was lucky to find me an airstrip."

"A small private airport?" Simon asked.

"Worse. It was a secret military airport."

"Why was it worse?"

"They refused me permission to land. I landed anyway."

"What did they say?"

"There was this British guy there, Sir Cecil something. Red hair, red mustache, looked mean. He comes up to me and says, you damn Yank, what the hell do you think you're doing here? And I told him, look, Idi Amin is holding my engineer and I need to get him the hell out of Uganda. He says, that's outside your abilities, you damn Yank, and I said, *whoa* boy, hold on, I'm from Texas, I'm not a damn Yank!"

I stood up and checked the IV again. I straightened Dell's arm and the blood flowed faster.

"Don't bend your elbow, the IV's positional," I warned.

"We got to talking and had food and a couple drinks. Actually became friends! Turns out, the guy was born in Scotland but was raised in Kenya. Spoke the local lingo like a native! The British ruled Kenya, you know, and he was their intelligence chief, or at least someone pretty high up. There had been a big rebellion against the British and it was pretty nasty."

"The Mau Mau," Simon said.

"That's right, the Mau Mau. The Mau Mau guys were pretty violent, and they hid out in the jungles. The villagers were terrified of them because if you didn't join them, well, the Mau Mau would come and cut your head off and drink your blood and stuff like that. The Mau Mau leader was hiding out in the jungles and this guy, Sir Cecil, and his boss, Lord Ian Something, tracked him down by sending locals pretending to be Mau Mau recruits deep into the jungles and gathering intel. So he figured out where this Mau Mau leader was hiding out and managed to surround him. Big bloody battle, with airstrikes and all. Anyhow, right after they finally capture this guy, guess what?"

Dell looked at me and winked.

"He gets a call that some British Royal Princess is visiting

Nairobi and would like to see him so would he please clean up and scrub all the dirt and blood off and put on a fresh uniform and comb his hair and come to Government House and meet the Royal Princess!"

"Do you mean a real British Princess?" Simon asked.

"Yes! Some British royal, I don't remember who, exactly. Anyhow, he captures this big leader, chief of the whole rebellion, then gussies up and meets the Princess, kisses her hand and all and talks about the weather and then goes back to the lock-up and interrogates Mr. Big!"

"All in one day?" Simon said, incredulously.

"Yes, all in one day! He told me about it!"

"That's amazing!" Simon said.

"He said the RAF - Royal Air Force - attacks were kind of useless in the jungle, but he did get to meet several bush pilots. He said he would find me the best bush pilot and would send him to go get my man. But I couldn't go, it was too risky."

"He arranged it? Out of friendship?" I asked.

Dell laughed.

"No, Doc, for money. We paid through our nose! Heck, we lost so much money there we were lucky to stay in business!"

"So what happened to your man in Uganda?" Simon asked.

"Sir Ian found me a pilot and he gave me one of his best guys. He got them both into Ugandan uniforms and painted a Ugandan logo on the outside of my plane. Next Sunday, we tried it again. So his pilot takes off, lands near Kinshasa, and guess what? Fletch had gone to the wrong spot. So the pilot comes back without him."

"How did you communicate with your guy, Fletch?" I asked.

"Sir Ian found a contact in the British High Commission. We got the information to Fletch and tried again, the next Sunday. Third time! The pilot landed, Fletch got on, but suddenly his Ugandan guards showed up. Took out their tommy guns and stopped the plane. Wanted to see their papers."

"What papers?" Simon asked.

"Transfer papers, saying that they could hand Fletch over to the Ugandan Air Force, because that's what they thought they were doing."

"But did they have any papers?" Simon asked.

"Nope. But the pilot was one sharp cookie. So the pilot signs his fake flight manifest and his fuel bill, his registration papers, and a couple other useless papers that happen to be in the plane and hands the entire mess over and salutes them."

"Didn't they realize it was the wrong paperwork?" Simon asked.

"Pilot said, he figured if there was too much paper, no one would read it. He was right. They just took all the forms and saluted and stepped back."

"They let him take off? From the park?" Simon asked, astonished.

"Yep!" Dell laughed. "They let him take off. We got Fletch back!"

"So it ended well!" Simon said.

Dell shrugged.

"Not completely. Idi Amin was furious. He found out the real name of the pilot and some years later, put a bomb on his plane. Blew him to bits."

We were silent. Simon shook his head.

"Life's not fair, munchkins," Dell said.

I sat with Dell for another five minutes. Nothing had happened. I got up to leave.

"Dell, I'm going back to my clinic. I have a patient to see there. Simon will call me if there's any problem."

Dell held up his hand.

"Doc, I should have told you something. This morning I had some back pain," he said.

I paused.

"The pain started in my lower back and kind of went down to the left side, left groin. I figured, I've had this before, no big deal, it's a kidney stone."

"Why didn't you tell me this earlier?"

"It got better. And I didn't want you to cancel the transfusion. Two good reasons."

"Dell, you should have told me. I need to know these things in advance. Have you passed any blood in your urine?"

"Not this time. My urine sometimes gets red, but it didn't this time so that's why I figured it was no big deal."

"You need to check your urine again. If you are passing red urine, it could mean that you're having a transfusion reaction and destroying the red cells that we're giving you and passing pieces of red cells in your urine."

"You worry too much, Doc!" Dell said.

"Could you please get us a urine sample?"

"I don't feel like passing urine. And I want to get all the blood in before this IV blows. You said it was positional."

"If you are breaking down the blood we are giving you, it's no use to you. This could be very serious. We need to know, right now!" I insisted.

"Doc, like I said, I don't feel like I can pass any urine. Give me some water or coffee or something, and I'll try."

Simon ran to the nurses' station and reappeared with cups of water and coffee. Dell drank thirstily.

"When you're thirsty, even hospital coffee tastes good!" he said.

"Now more water," I insisted.

"You're a pushy little guy!" Dell declared, and gamely drank the water.

"I'm going upstairs, Simon," I said. "Be sure to check his urine and call me whatever the result. It's important!"

I walked into the clinic office. The manager, Tracy, called out.

"Hey, Dr. Mathur, you have a patient in Four."

"Thanks. Any others?"

"You have two more later this morning. They both just want you to refill their prescriptions till Dr. Becker returns."

"When is Karl coming back?"

"Next week. He's going to be here before you go to San Antonio for your immigration meeting."

"It'll be good to have Karl back. Too quiet without him."

"We're making the most of it," Tracy said. "Do you remember his fart machine?"

"Yes. He hid it in my clinic room for my very first patient. He set it off, luckily after I had finished talking. My patient told me, I know it's not you."

"That was sweet," Tracy said, tartly. "Did the patient ever come back to you?"

"Yes, she did. She said I was the best little Mexican doctor she had ever met."

Tracy smirked and went back to work.

"Good morning! I'm Dr. Mathur. Mrs. Hoofnagle?"

"That's me."

"Nice to meet you. I understand you are here because of neck pain. Is that right?"

"Well, I wouldn't really call it *neck* pain."

I sat down, facing her. She was a plump lady, short, with glasses and big hair. She wore stained jeans and a wrinkled blue shirt and smelled of sweat.

"So where is the pain?" I continued.
"Well, it starts in the neck but it's mostly in the shoulders."
"How bad is the pain?"
"Well, I wouldn't really call it pain."
"What would you call it?"
"More like an ache."
"How bad is it?"
"Pretty bad."
"On a scale of one to ten, ten being the worst pain you ever had, how bad is the pain?"
"Actually, I wouldn't call it pain."
I sighed.
"Okay, how bad is the ache?"
"Nine."
"Okay, a nine. Do you have this ache every day?"
"I wouldn't really say every day."
"Every other day? A few times a week?"
"No, I mean it happens at night."
"All right. How often does it happen at night?"
"Every night. At two a.m."
"How long does it last?"
"Until I do something to make it stop."
"What do you do to make it stop?"
"I have to get up and move around."
"So it goes on for several minutes?"
"I wouldn't say several minutes."
"An hour?"
"I wouldn't say an hour."
"Maybe two hours?"
"Yes. Maybe two hours."
"Okay, you're having a severe ache in your shoulders that happens every night at two a.m. and lasts two hours, or until you

get up and move around. Correct?"

"Yes."

"How long has this been happening?"

She shrugged.

"A month?" I asked.

"I wouldn't say a month."

I kicked myself.

"Then how long?"

"Three months."

"Getting better or worse?"

"I wouldn't say it's getting better."

"So it's getting worse."

"Yes."

"What have you done about it?"

"I'm Dr. Karl's patient so I called him."

"But he's not here!"

"I know. I called him in rehab."

"You called him in rehab?" I was incredulous.

"Yes. He ordered some labs and X-rays and scans right away. I got them done here with our lab. I know Tom Lightfoot. They were all fine. Then my daughter, who is a nurse in Fort Worth, got me in with an arthritis doctor and *she* ran a bunch of tests."

"Was everything normal?"

"I wouldn't say everything was normal."

I bit my lip.

"What was abnormal?"

"My cholesterol was high, the good and the bad."

"How high?"

"I don't know. She just said it was high."

"Is there a family history of heart attacks or strokes?"

"I'm adopted."

"Does anything make this ache better? Other than getting up and walking?"

"Sometimes I use oxygen."

"Oxygen?"

"My husband died of lung cancer. His oxygen is still at home."

"So you're short of breath?"

"Yes."

"Pretty short of breath?"

"I wouldn't say pretty short of breath."

I let it go.

"I read your chart before coming in and saw that you are on medicines for your thyroid and for high blood pressure. No allergies. No operations in the past?"

"Forgot to mention, C section."

I stood up and motioned.

"Please sit down on the examination table. I'm going to do a quick physical. You don't have to undress."

Her hands were rough and the nails black-rimmed. Her thyroid was normal. She had triangular yellow deposits on her eyelids. I listened carefully to her heart.

"Hear anything bad?" she asked.

"No."

"Then why are you still listening? Are you worried about my heart?"

"Yes," I admitted.

"Do you think it could be my heart?" she asked, concerned.

"It could."

"But it's an ache in my shoulders!"

"Women can have pretty odd presentations of heart pain," I explained.

"But heart problems get worse on getting up and moving

around and my ache gets better!"

"True."

I examined her neck and shoulders, and knees and ankles. I checked her muscle strength and reflexes. She chuckled as her feet shot forward.

"You know exactly where to hit!"

"You have good reflexes."

"Too good! Almost kicked my shoes off."

"Your sneakers are loose," I noted.

I helped her back to her chair. There was a knock at the door, and Simon stepped in, looking flustered.

"May I see you for a minute, Doctor?" he asked.

We stepped outside the room. Simon whipped out a plastic bag of orange liquid.

"Red! His urine's blooming red!" Simon burst out. "What do we do?"

"Stop the blood right away! Right now!"

"I did. I've got saline running to keep the IV going."

"Good. How's he doing?"

"Well, he's not too happy. He wants to finish the blood transfusion. He says his urine always looks like this when he's passing a stone."

"He could be passing a stone or he could be grinding up the red cells that we're transfusing and passing the fragments out in his urine!"

"You mean, he's having hemolysis?" Simon asked.

"Yes. We need to check his blood for hemolysis. We need Tom to check Dell's blood for LDH and haptoglobin, besides a CBC, stat!"

"Here's the other problem, Doctor," Simon sighed. "We can't do LDH in house. Or haptoglobin. They're send-outs. We have to send the blood to Abilene or Fort Worth for those tests."

"We can do a manual blood film, check the red cells," I said, thinking aloud. "But that's not confirmatory. Simon, we *need* to do the blood tests."

"So no more blood transfusion till then?"

"Correct."

"Dell is desperate. He wants to finish and go. Is there any other way to find out?" Simon asked.

I thought about my options.

"There is one way. Don't we have a centrifuge in the lab?"

"Certainly. I see them use it all the time."

"Then spin the urine. If it's kidney stones, then there should be intact red cells coming out in the urine, so if you spin the urine, the red cells should settle down and the urine should become clear."

"But what if there's hemolysis?"

"Then the urine won't clear up. The tiny fragments of smashed-up red cells don't settle down and the urine does not clear up. It will remain red."

"So if we spin the red urine and the plasma clears, then it's intact big red cells in the urine from kidney stones, and not tiny fragments or molecules of hemoglobin?"

"Exactly."

"So if we spin it and the urine clears, then it's kidney stones?"

"Yes."

"And if it remains red then it's a transfusion reaction?"

"Exactly!"

"We can do that! He has another unit of blood so he really needs to know what's happening."

"Spin the urine. And send the blood to Abilene by courier to confirm."

"Will do."

Simon sped away. I went back to my patient.

"Thank you for your patience," I said.

Mrs. Hoofnagle waved.

"If it was me in the ER, I would have wanted you to attend to me. It's no problem."

I settled down in front of Mrs. Hoofnagle.

"I'm worried about your heart."

"My shoulders are hurting, not my heart!"

"But the work-up is completely normal! Your examination is normal. The X rays don't show any arthritis at all."

"Maybe I need a CT or MRI scan."

"If it was that subtle, it wouldn't bother you so much. Also, your cholesterol is high."

"That just started!"

"No, I think you have had high cholesterol for a long time. You have yellow patches on your eyelids."

She gasped and covered her face with her hands.

"Those yellow deals? I just forgot to put on my make-up!"

"Those are called xanthelasma, a collection of cholesterol under the skin. Those take years to develop."

"But my EKG was normal."

"The EKG was done when you were feeling okay. The time stamp says eight fifteen a.m. Your pain is present from two a.m. to four a.m. The EKG needs to be done when you're in pain."

"I wouldn't say pain."

"When you ache. At two a.m."

"How would I get an EKG at two in the morning?"

"Come to the ER. Your grandson can drive you."

"How do you know I have a grandson?"

"You're wearing his sneakers. You were probably working in the garden and your own shoes were muddy so you wore his. Shoes of a teenage boy, too big for your feet."

She smiled.

"How'd you know about my gardening?" she asked.

"Your fingernails have mud."

"You're right. I was in the yard. I had to get back in the house pronto for a phone call. Yes, Justin can bring me. But I'm feeling perfect right now, Doctor!"

"You need to come in at two a.m. to have an EKG when you're hurting. I'm going to send orders down to the ER, and I'm going to start you on a baby aspirin."

"You know who was calling me on the phone while you stepped out? It was Dr. Karl. You know what he said?"

I shook my head.

"He said, get in to see Dr. Sandi. Something's wrong, could be your heart."

I went home for lunch. Maya and the girls were outside in the backyard. We ate cucumber and cream cheese sandwiches and drank hot Darjeeling tea with cardamom. Priya and Anjali took turns on the swing.

"They have had more fun out of that little swing than anything else!" Maya smiled.

"Priya's wearing her cowboy boots with tassels," I noted.

"Never leaves home without them," Maya said.

"How's Anjali's hearing?"

"Better now. I plan to get her enrolled in early pre-K or pre-K at the school, so she can listen to other kids her age."

"You talk to her a lot."

"Yes, but she should hear other voices, other accents."

"She hears mine," I said, lightly.

Maya gazed at me.

"Not often enough," she said, slowly.

"I know I'm not home a lot," I admitted. "But it will get

better soon."

"How do you know?"

"Karl will be back next week," I said.

"Next week? That's great! Then you won't have to go to the hospital that much."

"That's what I thought."

"We have our immigration interview coming up in San Antonio, for our green cards."

"Karl will be here and he can cover for me."

"Let's go out for dinner together, before we go to San Antonio," Maya suggested.

"Good idea. We all need to have a nice dinner together."

"Not all of us. I'll get Billie to babysit."

"Just the two of us?"

"Just the two of us."

"Sounds romantic."

"We need to come up with a plan, a strategy."

Maya stood up abruptly and walked to the swing.

Simon called me at home.

"The urine cleared up!"

"Good! So it's likely to be kidney stones and not a transfusion reaction. Did you tell Mr. Clawsom?"

"Yes."

"What did he say?"

Simon chuckled.

"He said, I told you so."

"He wasn't impressed by my use of local technology to solve a critical issue?"

"No."

"In India, we call this jugaad."

"Jugaad?"

"Yes, jugaad. The art of making things happen with limited resources."

"We definitely have limited resources, Doctor. So can I continue the transfusion?"

"No, it's not safe. Get the labs done in Abilene and call me with the results. Store the blood in the lab refrigerator."

"He's not going to like it."

"It's safer. Just wait a few hours."

"Hold on, he's here. I'll tell him."

There was a pause. I heard some laughing in the background.

"He says he wants it now, he wants to have it all right now, or he won't pay for any of it!" Simon relayed.

"Tell him, that's what the bishop said to the actress."

There was another pause, with more laughter.

"He says he's going to forgive you this time," Simon concluded.

We resumed the transfusion at ten that night.

"I'm sorry, the lab in Abilene messed up and we had to send another sample of your blood and then the blood bank wanted to repeat the tests on the second unit," I explained.

"But everything was okay," Simon added.

"So all this was for nothing?" Dell asked, in mock anger.

"Yes. We did it to irritate you," Simon said.

"It worked. You irritated the heck out of me!"

"We're British. We follow protocol," Simon defended.

"Waste of time. Should have been done with this hours ago."

"At least we got to hear your story," Simon offered.

Dell grunted. Simon flushed the IV line and Dell settled back down. I repeated the IV Benadryl and Solumedrol.

"If you Brits were so smart we wouldn't have had to bail you out so many times!" Dell growled.

Simon nodded.

"Her Majesty's Government has made a few errors over the years, I will admit that," Simon conceded.

"A few errors!" Dell guffawed. "More like dozens of first-class disasters!"

"We don't want to make a medical error, Bill," I interrupted. "Let me know if you feel anything."

"I feel irritation. I feel tired. I feel hungry!" Dell answered.

"Let me know if you have itching, a rash, chest pain or difficulty breathing."

Dell turned to look at me and paused.

"Let *me* know if you need me to write you a letter of support," he said.

I froze.

"Everyone knows you have to go to the immigration interview in a couple of weeks. Old man Rutherford was so pissed with you. Says you didn't treat his wife right, he may have sent a letter to the INS saying, hey, whatever you do, don't let this guy in," Dell said, casually.

I looked at Simon. Simon shrugged helplessly.

"I didn't say anything!" he swore.

"So if you would like me to help you, send a letter of support, just tell me."

I thought for a minute.

"Please do. Please write a letter of support for me," I said, quickly.

"Then I will do it."

"Thank you."

"I'll do it because I want to do it, not just because you asked me. And thank you for seeing my neighbor."

"Who's your neighbor?"

"Lucille Hoofnagle."

"I can't discuss other patients. But you're welcome."

"She said she has shoulder pains and you think she's fixing to have a heart attack!"

"I can't comment on another patient."

"Don't be scared!"

"I'm not scared. I'm being cautious."

"You're as scared and cautious as a long-tailed cat in a room full of rocking chairs! Go home to that sweet family of yours! I'm going to be just fine," Dell laughed.

"I'll wait a little."

Dell wagged his finger at me.

"Doc, you spend way too much time in the hospital. You need to spend less time here, more time at home. Your family needs you."

I nodded.

"I'm going to see a couple of patients I admitted today and check on them."

"Then head home right after that, Doc."

"I will check on you too, and then head home."

"You're a good man, Doc. But you need to go home."

There was an EKG waiting for me the next morning. I looked at it and jumped.

"Mrs. Hoofnagle's EKG! It's positive! There are changes!" I cried.

"Here's another one after her pain settled," Simon said, and handed me another.

"That one's normal. So she was having angina!"

"So it would seem. I concur, Doctor."

"Why didn't you call me?"

"It was three in the morning and she told me not to wake

you up"

"What?"

"Mrs. Hoofnagle told me you needed time to sleep and be at home. She said she had been having this pain for a month."

"She needs to see a cardiologist right away! Let's refer her to Dr. Leverton in Abilene."

"That's what she wanted. I called Dr. Leverton's office, faxed them both EKGs, and they gave her an appointment for ten a.m."

"Ten a.m. today?"

"Yes, Doctor."

"Does she know?"

"She's on her way there right now. Grandson's taking her."

I sat down and reviewed the case in my mind.

"Women do have atypical presentations," I said aloud.

Simon handed me the paperwork.

"You were right, Doctor," he said.

I completed my notes and handed them back.

"Some news from San Antonio. Not good. Brian, the young man with burns, went into septic shock. He's in the ICU."

"How bad is it?"

"Sally said he doesn't look good."

"Will they let me see him if I go to the Air Force Hospital?"

"When you go to San Antonio for your green card interview?"

"Yes."

"I don't know. If Sally calls again, I'll ask her."

"So she called to update us?"

"Actually, she wanted the words of that poem. I dictated it to her."

That poem. I remembered the night.

"My Love is Like a Red, Red Rose?" I asked.

Simon turned away.

"Yes," he said, quietly. "The most beautiful of all his poems, I think. She liked it a lot."

I nodded.

"She said she wanted it to be the last thing he ever heard," Simon added, "in case, you know."

I thought of the young man and his fiancee, and it seemed impossible.

"I can't believe it!" I protested. "I'm sure he'll pull through!"

Simon coughed and paused. He said nothing.

"Based on my years of experience, I feel that he's going to make it," I said, with conviction.

Simon looked out the door.

"She really thinks Brian might die tonight," he said, and left the room.

CHAPTER 18

STRATEGY

I finished rounding on my in-patients and wheeled the cart back to the nurses station. I wrenched out a stack of charts and sat down. I wrote and reviewed my notes, signed them, and replaced the charts. I checked with the nurses to make sure that I hadn't missed any orders. After that, I called home. Maya and I were going to have dinner together, just the two of us.

"Maya, I was just calling to confirm. I've made reservations for us to have dinner at Bonnie's at six-thirty. Did the baby-sitter show up?" I asked.

"Yes, I'm with Billie right now. Priya and Anjali are finishing dinner and then Billie is going to take them to the drawing room and will read to them."

"Did they get their chocolate-chip cookies?"

"One each, as promised. Have you seen all your patients?" she asked.

"I've seen all my in-patients. I do have one patient to see in the ER, but it shouldn't take long. I wanted to tell you that, for once in my life, I'm going to be on time."

There was a pause.

"You may get delayed," Maya said, quietly. "That case in the ER will probably take an hour."

"No, I don't think so. I'm sure I can manage."

"What's the patient's problem?" Maya asked.

"Uncontrolled blood pressure. Shouldn't be too difficult, really," I answered.

There was a longer pause.

"I'll bring a magazine," Maya declared.

"No, I won't be late," I promised. "I'll see you at Bonnie's at six-thirty. You won't need the magazine."

I walked briskly to the Emergency Room. Simon looked up in surprise.

"They didn't tell you?" he asked.

"Tell me what?"

"That the patient left?" Simon said.

"She left? Why?"

"She wanted to see Dr. Becker."

"But Dr. Becker won't be here till tomorrow!"

"I told her that. She said she would wait and see him in the clinic tomorrow."

"What about her blood pressure?"

"Rather high, one hundred and ninety by ninety five."

"That's very high! Did you tell her it was serious?"

Simon nodded.

"Yes, of course, Doctor. I told her it was very high, dangerously high."

"High enough it could cause a heart attack or stroke?" I persisted.

"Yes, I believe I mentioned that."

"Did you tell her I was in the hospital?"

"I did."

I walked to the window and looked out at the parking lot. Three trucks, my red Corolla, and nothing else.

"Was she concerned that there would be a long wait?" I wondered.

"No, I don't think she was worried about having to wait a long time for you."

"She still left? I don't understand," I persisted.

"She said she wanted to see Dr. Becker," Simon repeated,

speaking slowly and deliberately.

I was irritated.

"You said she understood the risks. Did she sign a form saying she was leaving against medical advice? The AMA form?" I asked, sharply.

"She refused to sign an AMA. Said her insurance wouldn't pay if she did that."

"But she did exactly that!" I protested.

Simon sighed and shrugged.

"Doctor, she was determined to go and she popped out when I wasn't looking. I was distracted. My abject apologies."

"What were you doing?" I snapped.

Simon waved an envelope.

"Sally Nieves came by," he said quietly.

"Yes, I remember Sally. How is Brian?"

Simon shook his head and handed me the envelope.

"He didn't make it. Sally came by to thank us and left this envelope."

I was stunned.

"He died?" I gasped.

Simon nodded.

"He *died*? How could that happen? He was so young! He was strong! The burns were bad but not that bad!"

Simon nodded silently.

"The burns were *not* that bad! No! How could he have *died*?" I repeated, angrily.

Simon said nothing. I was bewildered.

"I just don't understand. He was young, had some burns, severe but not critical, not that extensive. It doesn't make sense. How could he have *died*?"

Simon gazed at me blankly. I paced the room.

"I just don't understand it. Did Sally say anything about it?

What happened?"

"She just said that Brian became septic and went into shock three days after reaching San Antonio. He was really bad the first night, then got better, came out of ICU, was sitting up and talking and eating, so she went to a motel to sleep. The next morning he was back in the ICU and had a cardiac arrest."

I sat down and exhaled.

"I just can't believe it. He looked so good when he left. We gave him Rocephin and plenty of fluids. We did everything they asked us to do!"

"We did," Simon agreed.

I looked at the envelope. It had been folded over several times.

"It's not addressed to anyone," I said.

"She just left it here," Simon said.

I ripped it open and scanned the crumpled paper.

"My love is like a red, red rose," I read aloud. "It's the first stanza of your poem!"

"It's Burns' poem!" Simon was surprised. "That's the Burns poem I wrote out for her when they were here! She returned it?"

I examined the paper closely.

"No, it's more interesting than that. It's not your handwriting. Also, there's a mark in the upper right corner, it says LAFBH."

"What does that mean?" Simon wondered.

"Probably Lackland Air Force Base Hospital. So *she* wrote it while he was in hospital, probably when you dictated it over the phone. She wrote it for him because she liked it."

"How do you know *he* didn't write it for *her*?" Simon asked.

"His right hand was burned, remember? He couldn't sign his papers or hold his license. Sally had to hold up his expired driver's license."

"That's right."

Simon sat down and looked at me. His face was flushed and he avoided looking at me.

"I feel hollow and guilty. I feel awful. I feel like crying out loud, but I can't. Just can't, but all hot inside," he said.

I nodded. There was silence for several minutes.

"It hurts a lot. We shouldn't take this personally, but we do. Very personally. Every failure hurts badly," I said.

"Do you remember your failures more than your successes?" Simon asked.

I thought about that.

"Actually, my failures are seared into my brain. I never forget them," I said. "I usually forget about the successes."

"Does it not cripple you?" Simon wondered.

"No," I answered, "but it definitely makes me modest."

Simon picked up the patient chart and handed it to me.

"You need to co-sign it. It's for the patient who fled."

I read the note. It said *Patient left before being seen. Patient said she preferred to see Dr. Becker tomorrow. She understands the risks of waiting.* I co-signed and handed the clipboard back.

"It's her funeral," I said, bitterly.

Simon looked at me with surprise.

"You're upset that the patient left?" he asked.

"Yes."

"Because she could have serious medical problems?"

"Yes."

Simon paused and smiled.

"And a tiny bit, very tiny, maybe very, very tiny bit upset she wanted to see Dr. Becker, and not you?" he asked.

I hesitated and thought about it.

"Yes," I admitted.

I stood up to leave.

"You're rather smartly turned out today," Simon noted.

"Blazer and tie and all! Something special?"

"Taking Maya out for dinner."

"Anniversary?"

"No. Just an evening together. No occasion."

I stuffed the envelope in my coat pocket. I walked to the door.

"Rough, isn't it? I didn't think we would lose Brian," Simon said.

"I thought you would say, bloody awful business, but keep a stiff upper lip. That would be the British thing to say."

"Like flies to wanton boys are we to the Gods, they kill us for their sport," Simon lamented.

"Excuse me?" I paused at the door.

"Just like boys kill flies on a whim, carelessly, whenever they desire, the Gods just kill us too, without reason, just for fun," Simon explained, helpfully.

I nodded.

"The Americans have a shorter version," I said.

"And that is?" Simon wondered, disbelieving.

"Shit happens," I quoted.

I reached the steak house early. We had decided to come in separate cars in case I had to go back to the hospital. The steak house was a log cabin fronted by a porch, with colorful lights strung around the door and windows. The smell of roasting meat jolted me in the parking lot, and I immediately remembered Brian. I struggled to put those memories aside. I had to focus on the task ahead: the strategy for the interview. We had an interview with the immigration authorities in San Antonio, and I knew there were hurdles in our way. I parked and walked up to the front door. I smelled barbecue and raucous perfume as I stepped inside.

"Welcome, Doc! Where's your pretty wife?" The owner, Bonnie Bail, a tall woman with grey hair and half-moon glasses, hugged me.

"Maya is on her way. She was getting the girls squared away with the babysitter."

"I know she likes fish. I've got delicious catfish! I got some shrimp, too, just in case!"

"Thank you, Bonnie."

"Got you a nice table right here in the middle. Close to the salad bar."

"Maya loves salad," I nodded. "This will work nicely. How's that rash doing?"

Bonnie smiled widely and showed me her wrists.

"All gone! Healed up like a charm! I guess you were right, it was that nickel jewelry!"

"I'm delighted that you're better," I said.

Bonnie hesitated.

"Doc, I got a favor to ask you. Would you see my grandson? I understand if you say no."

I sat down and looked up at her.

"What's the problem?"

"He's a teenager, *that's* the problem. Actually, he just told me about a rash on his arms. Will you take a look at it?"

"Sure. Bring him to the clinic tomorrow."

Bonnie shook her head.

"Won't go to the clinic. But I got him right here. You mind taking a quick peek at it?"

I thought for a minute. I glanced out at the parking lot. There was no sign of Maya.

"If I can see him before Maya gets here," I said. "I want to clear my mind and focus for a few minutes."

Bonnie scanned the room.

"Where is he? I bet he just went to the restroom, dang it!" she said, and slammed her jug of ice tea down. "What is it with that boy?"

"Remember, I can't see him once Maya gets here. I need to talk to Maya about a couple of important things."

"I'll bet. Like your green card interview in San Antone? With immigration?"

I was taken aback.

"And of course, Doc Becker is back and he's going to take all his patients back, so not so much left for you, kind of got your snout pushed out of the trough, I guess," Bonnie said, nodding with concern. She glanced at me.

"What?" she asked. "Did I say something wrong?"

"No," I admitted. "That's exactly what I want to talk about. Sometimes I'm surprised how obvious things are to everyone."

"My daughter's an LVN, works in the hospital," Bonnie shrugged. She spied a young man leaving the restroom.

"Bless his heart, there he is! I'll get him!" she said, and scuttled off. She returned with a scowling teenager.

"Doc, this is my grandson Garrett," she said, proudly.

Garrett was short and thin, with light brown hair and green eyes. He took off his hat and offered a hand.

"Nice to meet you," I said, and shook his wet hand.

"Wet because I washed," he explained.

"I'm glad it wasn't on account of something else," I said.

Garrett grinned.

"What else could it be?" he dared.

"Blood. Phlegm. Saliva. Some others I can't name I'm in your grandmother's restaurant."

"I bet!" he chuckled.

"So what's up, Garrett?"

"I got this crazy little rash. Bunch of little bumps. Really hurts."

He sat down and pulled up his shirt sleeves. There were tiny blisters on the back of the elbows, and the skin was red. There were straight black lines in between and around the rash.

"Does it itch?"

"Powerful itches!"

"Is there a rash anywhere else?"

"No. Just on the back of my elbows. Had it on my knees a couple years ago."

"So you've had this problem for at least two years. Any other medical problems?"

"No, sir."

Bonnie placed a hand on his shoulder.

"Tell him about your diarrhea, son."

Garrett flushed.

"Nothing to be embarrassed about. He's a doctor. You can tell him."

Garrett looked away. Bonnie shook his shoulder.

"You just came out of the restroom! That's the fourth time today, that I've seen you go number two!"

Garret squirmed.

"Nana, don't say that! Yes, okay? I got diarrhea! Jesus, Nana!"

"Don't blaspheme, Garrett!"

Garrett groaned.

"Okay, So you've had diarrhea and this rash for at least two years. Right?"

"Right."

"More than two years?"

"Yeah."

"Five years?"

"Could be."

"Since you were a kid?"

"Forever."

"Why didn't you just say that?" Bonnie asked, irritated.

"He didn't ask," Garrett shrugged.

"No heart or lung problems?"

"Nope."

"Any other medical problems?"

"Nope.

"Tell the truth now!" Bonnie insisted

Garrett scowled.

"He was anemic. But I got him fixed! Made him eat steak for a month and his anemia went away!"

"It came back. I'm with anemia again."

"What? Why didn't you tell me?" Bonnie was upset.

Garrett shrugged.

"No operations ever?"

"No."

"Any illnesses run in your family?"

"Don't know much about my dad. He kind of abandoned us."

"Are brothers and sisters healthy?"

"One younger brother and sister. I'm the oldest."

"Who's the tallest?"

"Little brother."

"And your sister?

"She's taller than me, too."

"So you're the shortest?"

He grimaced.

"Yeah," he admitted, "I'm the runt."

"That could mean that you've had poor absorption of food for many years that affected your growth. If you're anemic, that usually means you are low in blood. My best guess is that you have celiac disease."

"What's that?"

"That's a disease where you're very allergic to gluten, a protein in wheat. So whenever you have anything made with wheat, like bread, you have a severe allergic reaction in your intestine. The intestinal lining breaks down, the reaction is so bad. Then you can't absorb iron, so you become anemic."

"And you can't absorb food so you're shorter," Bonnie nodded.

"Right. That could be why he's always been shorter than his siblings."

"What's this got to do with the rash?" Garrett asked.

"Your immune system gets all messed up. It produces an antibody that damages the intestine that stops you from absorbing food but sometimes that antibody can also attack the skin and cause tiny blisters."

Garrett inspected his elbows.

"The rash is called dermatitis herpetiformis. It will go away if you avoid foods with wheat."

"Then how did he have it when he went hunting with his friends?" Bonnie asked. "They lived on turkey and venison and potatoes. That's all there was in my little cabin."

I turned to Garrett.

"Did you have any beer?" I asked.

He grinned.

"God forgive us!" Bonnie cried.

"Anyhow, stop all wheat products and you'll get a lot better. You should see an improvement in a couple of weeks."

"Will I get taller?"

"Boys often keep growing into their late teens so yes, you could."

"Best news I heard all month!" he whooped.

I spied Maya in the parking lot.

"My wife's here. I can't talk to you anymore. I have important things to discuss with her," I said.

"You should've got her some roses, a pretty young thing like that deserves roses. Shame on you!" Bonnie said.

"I should have," I admitted, "but it's too late now. Next time."

Bonnie and Garrett retreated.

"Thanks, Doc! Let me see if I can get you some roses for your pretty little bride!"

I went to the door and greeted Maya and brought her to the table.

"I always think of you having your job interview here," Maya smiled.

"Right next to the sign."

"The sign that says, *I wasn't born in Texas but got here as fast as I could.* Yes, I know."

"That's the meeting where they decided to offer me the job."

"And here we are, almost two years later."

I nodded.

"I wanted to spend a quiet evening with you. Doesn't look like I made a wise choice. It's pretty noisy here."

"It's fine, it's fine."

"At least the food's always good."

"It was this or Dairy Queen, right?" Maya said.

"Right. Difficult decision."

Maya glanced at the menu.

"Do they still have fish?"

"Sure. And there's a decent salad bar."

"Billie was running a few minutes late. She has the girls coloring their books and then she's giving them cheese pizza."

"Great! Billie is just the right person. She looks like a grandmother, with the white hair and a big smile and round glasses."

Bonnie greeted Maya and they hugged.

"I know what you want, pretty lady. No need to ask. Tilapia, blackened, with rice and asparagus. What about you, Doc?"

"I'll have the same."

"Ice tea for the both of you?"

"Yes."

"Help yourselves to the salad bar. Be right back with some fresh bread and butter."

The salad bar was in the center of the room. As we walked back, I heard a call.

"Hey, Doc! It's Dell Clawsom!"

I turned. Dell and his wife Louise got up and introduced themselves to Maya.

"We got ourselves an Indian princess here!" Louise declared. Maya blushed.

"Thank you! It's nice to meet you."

"Don't let us interrupt you! Enjoy your dinner. I'll catch up with Doc later," Dell said.

"Dell told me about your helping him with the blood transfusion," Louise said. "He really liked you!"

"Glad to help. Dell, call me and I'll set up a follow up lab test."

"Why?"

"To make sure that your blood count isn't dropping."

"Why would it drop, Doc?"

"In case you're losing it somewhere, or you're not making blood."

"That's why I'm here eating steak! Lots of red meat to get iron and get my blood back up again!"

"Call me. We still need to check."

Dell nodded and returned to his dinner.

We sat down and sipped iced tea.

"You said we all have to go to San Antonio," Maya said.

"We have interviews for the green cards. Yours and Priya's are just formalities, but mine is a big deal. They like to ask a lot of questions."

"Did the hospital's lawyer go over things with you?"

"Yes. There's one thing I'm worried about."

"The letter Mr. Rutherford wrote? About his wife?"

"Yes. You remember I told you, she had a stroke and everyone wanted me to give her that special medicine?"

"The medicine to dissolve the stroke?"

"The medicine to dissolve the *clot* that caused the stroke. Yes. But I couldn't, because she was bleeding from a stomach ulcer. There could have been severe bleeding, and she could have died from the bleeding. That kind of bleeding can't be controlled."

"Is there an antidote to the medicine that dissolves the clot?"

"No. No antidote. If you start bleeding, you're going to bleed to death."

"What did the specialists in Abilene say to you?"

"They agreed with me. But Mr. Rutherford didn't. He was furious!"

"And he wrote to the immigration lawyer and the immigration service to complain about you?"

"Yes."

"Don't you have letters from the specialists to say that you made the right decision?"

"Yes. But the hospital's lawyer said that he read Mr. Rutherford's letter and it was very strong and emotional."

Maya ate her salad and thought.

"So what does he advise you to do?" she asked, after a minute.

"He says, the immigration officer may ask me if there's anyone who opposes my request for permanent residence. He says I should say no."

"But you know that Mr. Rutherford opposes you!"

"Well, technically speaking, I have not *seen* the letter. I *believe* it to be true but I don't really *know* for sure."

"That sounds like a lawyer's answer to me," Maya said, flatly.

"The lawyer said, just avoid the whole issue."

Maya was incredulous.

"By *lying* about it?" she said.

"Is it really lying?"

"It sounds like you're lying."

"That's what the hospital lawyer advised," I shrugged.

We ate our salads silently.

"We've come so far," I said. "I hate to mess it all up with this one thing."

"So you're going to say no, I don't know anyone who opposes my application?"

"That's what I'm asking you. Should I do what the lawyer says or not?"

"You should say, there is a resident of Hotspur who is angry with me for not giving his wife a blood thinner. I did not give it because it would have caused severe bleeding. I have specialists to back me up," Maya advised, firmly.

"Just tell them everything?" I whimpered.

"Yes. Tell them everything."

"Our lawyer needs to get depositions from the specialists in Abilene. That could take months."

"So let it take months."

"But that means I don't have anyone to back me up at the interview."

"Let them hear you out, just tell them the whole story. Be

honest and open."

"The lawyer said not to do that. He said they would believe a citizen over a foreigner every time."

Bonnie brought two steaming platters with grilled fish, buttery rice, and asparagus. Several heads turned and nodded.

"Watch out now, it's hot!" Bonnie warned.

"It looks wonderful!" Maya exulted.

Bonnie turned to me.

"Doc! His mom put him on a gluten free diet for two weeks! Rash didn't get better!"

Maya looked confused.

"The rash takes several weeks to go away. Two weeks wasn't enough time. Get the labs done for celiac disease after he's been on a regular diet for at least two weeks, otherwise the tests turn negative on a gluten free diet," I insisted.

Bonnie nodded and departed.

"The immigration lawyer called me today," I said.

"We have the hearing day after tomorrow, right?" Maya asked.

"He wanted to know my strategy. If the immigration officer asks me, do you know anyone who objects to my application for a green card, should I say yes or no?"

"I can't believe you. After all this, you're still wondering? After Rutherford yelled at you in the parking lot!"

"I know. But the lawyer says, leave it alone. Maybe they don't have anything from him."

"But your lawyer said he read the letter! You know someone opposes you!"

I nodded.

"So how can you deny it?" Maya was concerned.

"He says, don't give them any ammunition. It's not likely that he did anything about it, he said. So just let it slide," I said, miserably.

Maya ate slowly and considered it.

"Seems wrong to me," she said, eventually.

"That was my question. Should I say no, and let it slide, because the INS doesn't know what happened in the parking lot?"

"I told you, it doesn't sound right."

"They *may* have nothing from him."

I finished eating in a hurry. I leaned forwards.

"If they have nothing, and I volunteer this information, they might start an investigation."

Maya shrugged.

"It might delay our green cards."

"It might."

"It could mess it up badly."

Maya looked at me evenly. She was unmoved.

"This is a big deal. We're waiting on our green cards. It affects our entire family. We could be stuck for years," I pleaded.

"How come?"

"The new policy is to change J visas to H visas and then to green cards years later."

"I understand. It could get dragged out. It would cost the hospital more," Maya said.

"The hospital is still low in cash. If my application gets dragged out, they may run out of cash."

"Then *we* can pay him."

"That's thousands of dollars!"

"If that's what it takes, spend the money!"

"Do we really want to get into all this mess? Could we not just avoid it?"

"It's dishonest."

I sighed.

"That's what I thought you'd say," I admitted.

"So you were questioning whether to tell the truth?"

"Sometimes it's simpler to be economical with the truth."

"This is what worries me about you and about doctors. You think that you can say what you want and get away with it. That everyone holds you in such regard they wouldn't question you. That you can't be questioned."

"No, I don't feel that way."

"Doctors always feel superior to everyone."

"I don't."

"Why are you different?"

"Because I'm married to you."

Maya smiled.

"But you have to remember, you're a family man. Not just a doctor."

I nodded.

"Remember us, too," Maya said, "we need your time. You need to be a husband and a father, not just a champion of a doctor."

We finished our meal. Bonnie was busy so I went to the counter and paid. Maya left and I headed to my car.

"Doc! Hey, Doc!" Bonnie called out.

I turned. Bonnie scrambled down the steps with a bouquet of roses.

"Dell Clawsom got these specially delivered from the Moral Floral. For you to give to your wife!"

"That's very kind!" I forced a smile.

"He said you know a poem about red roses. Maya might ought to hear it!" Bonnie huffed.

"Well, she's already gone home. I'll give it to her at home. Tell Bill, thanks a lot."

"You bet!" Bonnie beamed. She hugged me and left.

I waited for her to go back inside and let my face cloud over. I put the roses on the back seat and tossed my blazer on top of them. I drove home upset and confused, with mounting dread about the upcoming interview in San Antonio.

CHAPTER 19

THE GREEN CARD INTERVIEW

The main waiting area in the INS building was busy. Maya and I sat nervously and waited to be called. Priya and Anjali skipped around and gazed at other children and circled the vending machines. I checked and rechecked our papers, just in case I had left something vital in the car.

Maya heard them call our name. We sprung up and dashed to the window. I thrust the forms and affidavits at the official. She matched them against the information on her clipboard. She spoke without looking up.

"Wait here. We will call you for fingerprinting and photographs. All four need to be processed?"

"No, just three," I answered. "Anjali was born in Houston. She's a citizen by birth."

"Which one?" The official asked, not looking up from her clipboard.

"The little girl," I said.

"Okay, what about the other girl?"

"She's our older daughter, Priya. She does need to be fingerprinted and photographed."

"This woman is your wife?"

"Yes, Maya."

She shook her head and pushed my entire application back out.

"You should not have brought the little girl. *Only those that need to be processed.* It says so in capital letters on the letter we sent you."

"We don't have any family in Texas or anywhere to leave her."

"You should have left her at home."

"She's only five."

"You should have found a babysitter."

"We didn't know how long we might be in San Antonio. We could be here in San Antonio overnight, as our interview is at three p.m."

"You'll be done by four. Now we have a problem."

She was a short, plump lady with long, dark hair. She glared at the clipboard and shook her head again.

"You need to reschedule," she decided.

"No! Let's not do that. We've waited six months for this appointment!" I pleaded.

"You're not in compliance. *Only those needed for processing should attend.* Says so clearly."

"Yes, I understand. But please consider her age, and the fact that we live in Hotspur, which is four hours away."

"It's on the front page of your letter. Capitals. You need to re-schedule," she insisted. She pushed my application out. I grabbed it and slid it back.

A voice came from the far corner of the waiting room.

"Hotspur?"

I turned. A large man hunched over a water cooler, filling his carafe.

"We're from Hotspur," I announced.

The man ambled over. He was over six feet tall, weighed at least two hundred and fifty pounds, and had large dark-tinted glasses. His face and ears were covered with bright red spots.

"Hotspur, eh?" he repeated.

"Yes. Are you from Hotspur?" I asked, hopefully.

"Maybe," he answered. He looked at the four of us. I was in a dark suit and tie, Maya wore a light blue skirt and jacket, and Anjali was in a bright red frock with an American flag belt and matching barrettes in her hair. Priya defiantly sported a bizarre half-moon shaped red and green watermelon dress.

"Are you supposed to be a watermelon, mi hija?" he asked her.

"Yes," she answered, proudly.

"Why?" he asked.

"Because I like watermelons. It's my favorite dress. Look, the seeds are really buttons!"

He smiled at her, then looked up.

"What's the matter?" he asked the receptionist. She scowled.

"They brought their daughter who does not need to be processed. They were told to leave all unnecessary family at home. Now where do we leave the five-year-old girl? How do we take the others for processing?" the lady complained.

"I'm sure you told them that only those needing to be processed should come," the man said, soothingly.

"In capital letters, on the front page! How could it be clearer?" the lady said.

"Does Miss Watermelon need to be processed?" he asked.

"Yes."

"Okay, so who is the primary applicant?"

"I am," I said. "I'm Sandip Mathur."

"What are you here for?"

"For application for a green card."

"What's the status of little Miss Red Dress?"

"She's a U.S. citizen. She was born in Houston."

"So you're here for the permanent residency interviews. We need to interview the primary applicant and the dependents. Let's do this. You and little Miss American Red Dress come and sit in my office while your wife and Miss Watermelon get their work done. I'm doing some of the permanent residency interviews today. I think you're on my list. You two can sit in my office and do the interview, then you can go and get processed while I interview your dependents. Miss Red Dress can stay in my office," he proposed.

"No!" the lady cried.

The man gazed at her.

"She's unauthorized!" the lady protested.

The man shrugged.

"She's unauthorized!" the lady repeated, and pointed at Anjali.

"No, I'm Anjali!" Anjali bristled.

"They need to reschedule! That's the policy!" the lady declared defiantly.

But the man had already moved away.

"*Mr. Castillo!*" she pleaded.

Mr. Castillo waved his hand.

"Mr. Castillo! I will just reschedule them!"

Mr. Castillo shook his head and opened an office door. He turned and beckoned. The lady looked disgusted.

I saw my chance and seized it.

"Anjali, come with me! Maya, you and Priya get your fingerprinting! Anjali will be with me, then with you two!" I ordered. I lifted Anjali up and bolted, briefcase in hand.

The lady waved Maya and Priya towards another room. She looked disgusted.

I burst into Mr. Castillo's office and breathed again.

Mr. Castillo's office was a grey cubicle with a picture of President Clinton and a year planner. He sat behind a large metal desk with a glass top. A brass name-plate announced *Henry B. Castillo, Senior Examiner III*. He rummaged through a stack of files.

"Is the B for Bolivar?" I asked.

He didn't answer.

"I don't have your file," he declared. "Guess it's with Andy or Marisol."

My heart sank.

"But have a seat. I'll go see who has it. See if I can take it and do your interview."

"Thank you!" I said.

Mr. Castillo nodded and bustled out. I sat down on a metal chair and Anjali settled on the other. There was a moment of silence, then Anjali spoke.

"Can I have some chips?" she asked.

"We don't have chips," I answered.

"Mom put them in your bag."

She pointed to my briefcase.

"You sure?"

I opened my briefcase. Anjali dived in and retrieved a small bag. I noticed my cell phone had received a call from the hospital.

"You want some?" Anjali asked.

"No, thanks. Anjali, can you just stand at the door and tell me if the man is coming back?"

"Why?"

"Because I want to make a phone call, and we are not supposed to make calls from this office."

"Then why you doing it?"

"Because the hospital is calling. It might be an emergency."

Anjali slid off her perch and went to the door, munching chips.

I called the hospital.

"Hotspur Hospital!"

"This is Dr. Mathur. There was a call for me?"

"Yes, the lab wanted to get in touch with you. Hold on."

There was a pause.

"Lab. This is Tom."

"Tom, this is Dr. Mathur."

"Sorry to bother you, Dr. Mathur. I know you're in San Antone for your green cards. Had a critical on the lab you ordered for Mr. Dell Clawsom. Hemoglobin's six."

"The hemoglobin is six?" I asked, incredulously.

"Ran it twice. Six, six point one."

"That's crazy! I just transfused him!"

"Normal is twelve."

I bit my lip.

"Yes, I know the normal value. He needs blood. Is he having chest pain or difficulty breathing?"

"Don't know. He's sitting outside. Let me get him."

"I can't stay on the line! I'm here for my interview!"

But Tom had already set the phone down. I turned to look at Anjali. She was peering into the bag, scrounging for fragments.

"Anjali! Is the man coming?"

Anjali turned and shook her head.

"Hello, Doc!" Dell's voice squeaked.

"Dell! You don't sound good!" I said.

"Reckon losing half my blood has something to do with it?"

"Of course it does! Are you having some chest pain?'

"Nope."

"Are you short of breath?"

"If I get up and tend to something."

"Have you been passing blood with your bowel movements?"

"Nope."

Throwing up blood?"

"Nope."

"Passing black, tarry stools?"

"Well, yes. They're kind of dark."

"Are you taking iron or Pepto-Bismol?"

"Taking iron. On account of the anemia."

"Are your stools solid and dark grey-black, or liquid and jet-black?"

"They're solid, kind of dark grey."

"That sounds like iron and not blood. How many a day?"

"One a day. Regular as clockwork."

"Okay, so you're not bleeding. Any nose-bleeds?"

"No."

"No surgery or procedures since I last saw you?"

"Nothing since Burns Night."

I paused.

"Dell, your hemoglobin is critically low. You could have a stroke or a heart attack at any minute! You need to get to Abilene right away!"

"Can't you take care of it when you come back?"

"No, we need to take care of this right away!"

Dell sighed.

"Kind of guessed you were going to say that."

"You need to go to the ER and tell Dr. Becker what's going on. He can call Abilene and send you right away."

"Ambulance?"

"Yes!"

"Doc, they got their hands full. Old Rutherford's in there."

"Rutherford! What's he doing there?"

"Dying from a heart attack, by the looks of it."

My heart sank. *Maybe if I had been there, I could have helped him, maybe changed his opinion of me.*

"If you really think I should go to Abilene, I'll have Louise drive me there."

"Yes. You need to get up there."

"Alrighty then."

"Dell, how does it look for Mr. Rutherford?"

"I don't really know, Doc. From all the hollering and carrying on, doesn't look good. I reckon they're going to ship him to Abilene mighty fast!"

"I hope he makes it."

"Hope so too. Maybe give you another chance, to make good with him."

"Okay, Dell."

"Adios, Doc."

Anjali scuttled back.

"He's coming!" she sang out.

I disconnected and flung the phone inside my briefcase and snapped it shut. No one came.

"Just kidding," she grinned.

I was taken aback.

"You're trying to scare me!" I said, in mock anger.

"Yes!" she replied.

"It's not fair!" I protested.

"Life not fair, man-cub!" she giggled. We had watched *The Jungle Book* too many times.

Anjali sat down. I looked around the room. It was clean, smelled of air freshener and was well lit. There were no windows and only the one door. There were grey filing cabinets lining the wall behind the desk and a table with a coffee machine next to the door. The carafe of water was full and sat on a big red box of Folgers coffee.

Mr. Castillo entered, reading a file.

"So you're a doctor!" he noted.

"Yes, sir."

"Married, two daughters, born in India, worked in London, UK."

"Yes, sir."

"Then Medical Center Houston."

"Yes, sir."

"Then Hotspur!" he chuckled. "Hotspur! How big is it?"

"Five thousand in the town."

"Five thousand! You had millions in London and Houston!"

"Yes."

"How many doctors in Hotspur?"

"There were three. One went for back surgery and one had a heart attack."

"And one went to rehab," Mr. Castillo added.

"How did you know?"

"Oh, I know a little about Hotspur," Mr. Castillo smiled. "One went to rehab, right?"

"Yes," I admitted.

"So you were the only doctor in Hotspur?"

"For some months. But Dr. Becker just got back."

"And you had help from a part-time doctor?"

"That's correct."

Mr. Castillo opened my file and read the first page.

"Okay. Read this page and sign it," he said.

He leaned over and presented a folded piece of paper. He held onto the upper part.

"Just read and sign," he repeated.

"You can let go," I said.

"No. Just read that part. If it's correct then sign."

His fingers were tanned and stubby. He wore a wedding band and his nails had dark rims.

"I hear you fancy yourself as a good doctor," Mr. Castillo said.

I read the face sheet.

"This is our basic information, names, dates of birth, social security numbers and places we were born," I observed.

"Just check it."

I read it all again.

"It's correct."

"No spelling mistakes?"

"No."

"Hallelujah! It's a miracle!" Mr. Castillo declared, and yanked the page back.

"Some Indian names can be long and complicated," I conceded.

Mr. Castillo glanced over the next few pages of the file, then put it down.

"You fancy you're a *good* doctor?" He repeated.

"I try to be," I shrugged.

"Prove it," he said.

"What do you mean?"

"Prove it. Prove to me you're a good doctor."

I was at a loss. I looked at him blankly.

Mr. Castillo gazed back, his smile frozen.

"Prove to me you are what you say," he insisted.

"I can tell you about some interesting cases I saw in Hotspur," I offered.

"How would I know you're telling the truth about them?"

"You can call them."

"You think I have the time for that?"

I looked at Anjali. She rolled her eyes.

"Hurry up, Daddy!" she said. "I need to go to the bathroom!"

I looked at Mr Castillo. I saw the bright red spots covering his face and ears.

"You've been to the dermatologist. You've just had multiple skin cancers treated with Efudex cream."

Mr. Castillo blinked in surprise.

"Okay," he agreed, "but anyone can see that. What else?"

"You play golf. You like fixing old cars. You have a good marriage. And you have sleep apnea and high blood pressure."

Mr. Castillo paused, then laughed.

"You're right! But how the Sam Hill did you know all that?" he asked.

"You've got lots of skin cancers on your face. The commonest reason for that is being out in the sun a lot. In Texas, people stay *out* of the sun, except for one thing: golf."

"True. The old cars?"

"Black rimmed nails. In men, that means car repairs and in women, gardening."

"I got this '69 Chevy pickup," he admitted. "I'm working on it. It's my baby. But what about the rest?"

"You still have an old small wedding band. It's tight so you've had it for years and you've put on weight. Any woman that stays with you and lets you golf and fix cars is a really good wife!"

Mr. Castillo shook his head in disbelief.

"You're really going out on a limb."

"Maybe. But you have put on weight. Your belt has marks near the buckle and you've now got it all the way to the end."

"So I'm fat. So what? Does that tell you I have sleep apnea?"

"No, but your neck does. You're probably a size seventeen and a half or eighteen inch neck on your shirt size, right?"

"Eighteen."

"Anyone with a neck collar size over seventeen is at risk for sleep apnea. High blood pressure is very common with sleep apnea and being overweight."

There was a pause. Mr. Castillo stared at me with amusement.

"Are you trying to be Sherlock Holmes?"

I shrugged.

"Sherlock Holmes was based on a Professor of Medicine, Professor Bell, of Edinburgh, Scotland."

Mr. Castillo nodded.

"Makes sense. The guy who wrote that stuff, Conan Doyle, was a doctor."

"Yes, Professor Bell was his Professor in medical school."

"His medical professor was the basis for the Sherlock Holmes character?"

"Yes."

Mr. Castillo pondered that information.

"I need to go to the bathroom!" Anjali announced, loudly.

Mr. Castillo cleared his throat.

"Your application is in order, but there is one important issue."

"Yes, sir?"

"This is a very important issue. I want you to think carefully before you answer."

"I will," I promised. My heart began to race.

"We collect opinions from several citizens about your worthiness to be a permanent resident in the United States. We have obtained several favorable responses."

"I'm glad," I said.

"Do you know of anyone who might be opposed to your application?" Mr. Castillo asked, slowly and deliberately.

My mouth went dry. I didn't know what to say. Mr. Castillo leaned forwards.

"Is there any citizen of the United States, that you know of, who might object to your application?"

I looked away.

"Bathroom!" Anjali repeated.

"Doctor, I need your answer!"

I looked at Anjali desperately.

"I need your honest answer! Is there any U.S. citizen that you know of, who might oppose your application?" Mr. Castillo demanded to know.

I thought of Maya advising me at the steakhouse. *Tell the truth!*

"Doctor, could you please answer the question? Is there any U.S. citizen that you know of, who might oppose your application?"

I was beaten.

"Yes," I admitted.

Mr. Castillo was surprised.

"What did you say?" he asked.

"Yes," I repeated.

"You mean, yes, there is someone who objects to your application? Who is it?"

"There's a gentleman by the name of Rutherford who may object."

Mr. Castillo took off his glasses and wiped them with his cuff.

"Why?"

"Because I refused to give his wife a medicine to dissolve a blood clot that was causing a stroke."

"Why?"

"Because she had a bleeding ulcer. Giving her a clot-busting medicine called streptokinase would have resulted in massive bleeding. We would not have been able to stop the bleeding."

"Did Mr. Rutherford offer you a waiver for your actions? So you wouldn't be held responsible for the outcome of giving the dangerous medicine?"

"Yes, he did," I said, miserably.

"Yet you refused. Dio mio, what a decision! And you know what?"

I looked at him and shook my head.

"There was nothing like that in the file. But now that you've told me, I'm obliged to look into this issue."

My heart sank like a stone.

"You were so close! You would have had better luck by just not saying anything. This will delay the case about a year and triple the costs."

I felt nauseous. I desperately wanted to take my words back.

"You really messed this up!" Mr. Castillo chortled. "You really screwed up badly!"

I struggled to stay calm.

"So now what happens?" I croaked.

"We investigate this Mr. Rutherford and evaluate his claim. If there is sufficient evidence, then we will schedule a hearing for dismissal of your application."

"*Dismissal?* Dismissal of my entire application?" I was dumbfounded.

"Yes. Dismissal. You can always appeal. But it takes years. We're backlogged two years, three years at least."

I felt like throwing up. I thought of Maya and my daughters and realized I had gambled with their future. I plummeted into blackest despair.

"What can I do?" I said, helplessly. My throat dried up and my head throbbed. I fought back tears.

"Does your hospital have the money to keep fighting your case?"

"No."

"Do you have the money?"

"No."

"Then I guess it's over."

He stood up and stamped my file and signed it with a flourish.

I thought I would faint. Anjali pulled my sleeve urgently.

"Now! Bathroom!" she whimpered.

I stared at her in confusion. My vision blurred.

"Hey!" Mr. Castillo said.

I looked at him. He was grinning widely.

"I'm just messing with you."

"*What?*"

"Rutherford changed his mind and wrote a letter of *support* for you."

"What!"

"It's right here. Just like you said. First he was mad at you but the doctors in Abilene changed his mind."

"He changed his mind?"

"Yes, he did. And he said that you were a good son. I don't know why he said that."

"A good son?"

"I just approved your application, Doc. Just had to mess with you, you were being such a smart-ass. All that Sherlock Holmes and guessing about Bolivar!"

I was speechless.

"Now you better take that little daughter of yours to the bathroom while I hunt down your wife and daughter. Welcome to the United States!"

I snatched Anjali up. A familiar smell struck me.

"Or maybe it's you that needs to go to the restroom, Doc! I reckon I really got you there!"

Mr. Castillo guffawed and waddled out.

We shot off to the bathroom, slammed the door, and I finally breathed again.

An hour later the formalities were completed and we were all walking out. Maya waited until we were close to our car, then grasped my arm.

"Did he ask you the question?" she wanted to know.

"Yes."

"And what did you say?"

"I said, yes, there is someone who objects to my application."

"You said that?"

"Yes."

We strapped the girls into their car seats and settled down.

"So what did he say?" Maya asked.

"He said there was no objection from Mr. Rutherford. In fact, old Rutherford wrote a letter of support!"

"What?" Maya was incredulous.

"He sent them a letter supporting me and apparently said that I'm a good son."

"Where did that come from?"

"There's a little personal history. There's something else, some sad news."

"What?"

"Old Rutherford had a heart attack or something. I don't think he's going to make it."

Maya gasped.

"That's terrible! Poor, poor Patty!"

"I think we should send flowers," I suggested.

Maya nodded. We drove out of the parking lot in silence, and turned left on Evans Road. Soon we were on the I-10 freeway heading west.

"Now you can admit it," Maya said.

"What?"

"That I was right. It *was* better to tell the truth," Maya declared.

I turned to look at her in astonishment.

"Look in front! Drive carefully!"

I corrected myself.

"Just admit it, it's always better to tell the truth!" she repeated. She turned back to face the girls.

"Always tell the truth!" she instructed them.

I thought about it.

"Telling the truth can be complicated," I ventured.

"Only if you're weak," Maya countered.

"I was thinking of what Simon said. He said he didn't lie, he was merely economical with the truth."

Maya shook her head and turned to the girls again.

"The best strategy is to always tell the truth. *Always!* Remember that."

I smiled and drove on.

CHAPTER 20

THE KING RETURNS

I sat in Karl Becker's office, a converted corner room. He looked a lot thinner. His thick blond hair jutted out of a baseball cap that said *Big O's BBQ*. He wore a blue T-shirt and shorts and leaned back in his chair, his bare feet flapping on the desk in front of my face. The room reeked of raw onion-like sweat. Karl grinned.

"I heard you've been busy, Einstein," he said.

"Yes. You were gone and Dr. Bulent had a heart attack."

"Never knew he even had a heart, old Bulent."

"So I was the only one here. It got busy."

"What's this deal about us becoming a British hospital?"

"A reporter from Dallas showed up when Simon and I were working together. We have some British expats here, mostly women who married GIs after the war."

Karl shook his head.

"Ridiculous. This is Texas. You're almost American. Heck, one day you just might be Texan!"

"Right now I'm not American or Texan. I'm just tired."

"I'm back full time, man. I still got to go to Dallas for meetings once a week but that's just a day trip."

"Any particular day?"

"Usually Thursdays. Why?"

"Because Friday's would eat into the weekends. I would cover you, of course."

"I got to go today. Can you cover? I'll be back before midnight."

"Sure."

"Thanks, man."

He uncrossed his feet and sat up straight

"It's worse than cancer," he announced.

"What is?"

"Addiction. For years I had this beast sitting on my shoulders. I was terrified I'd get caught! I thought, what would everyone think? Everyone in my family, in my church, what would they say? Damn dopehead!"

Karl looked outside.

"Even when the shit hit the fan, I thought maybe I can keep this quiet. Respectable. Make it easy on my wife and kids. Know what happened?"

"Kind of."

"They put it in the paper. The paper! For everyone to read everywhere! Put my name there and everything! Don't know how my family handled it!"

"How was rehab?"

"Six months of being in a room with two other docs. Docs do drugs. A lot! One of the guys I was with, Andre, he did drugs and booze and porn. He was really bad. The other one, Oscar, was depressed. Not good, man, not good."

"Are you going to meet them in Dallas when you go for your weekly meetings?"

Karl laughed bitterly.

"Can't. Andre killed himself two days after rehab. Locked himself in his office and blew his brains out. Oscar doesn't answer my calls."

I was silent.

"That's why this is worse than cancer. So many relapses! So many suicides!"

"I had no idea it was that bad."

"Yeah, most docs think they're so superior. They think, I

can handle it because I'm the best of the best. Let me tell you something: we're the worst at diagnosing and treating ourselves. I guaran-damn-tee it!"

"So what are you going to do about it? So it doesn't happen to you?"

"You gotta take that addictive personality and channel it into something else. It doesn't just go away."

I was puzzled.

"What do you think I'm going to do, Einstein?" he asked.

It struck me.

"Running! You're taking up running. You've just been running!"

"Correct, Einstein! I'm going to run a half marathon and then a full marathon!"

"I wish I could do that."

"Why not?"

"I need to spend more time at home. Now that we've done the green card interview and now that you're back, I need to spend more time at home."

"Suit yourself. You know the hospital is going to pay us for covering the ER on weekends?"

"Yes," I said.

"I gotta make up for lost time and money. I'm going to do two weekends a month." Karl said.

"I'm going to stick to one weekend a month."

"You're losing money, man!" Karl said.

"I need to be home more," I said.

Karl nodded.

"Your call, man. I got three boys fixing to go to college, I need to provide. Your girls are still little."

"What happened to Rutherford?" I asked.

"He was dead before he got here. His wife had that stroke,

found him in the ranch somewhere way out, he was checking an oil well I guess. She gets on the phone and all she can say is shit and crap, so it takes forever to get the paramedics there. The clowns lose their way, even manage to hit a tree."

"So he was dead when he got here?"

"He had an agonal rhythm. There was heart electrical activity but no pulse, no meaningful activity, it had quit beating before the paramedics got there."

"So why send him to Abilene?"

"Sent him down to Abilene just in case. In case there was anything they could do for him. Heard he was pretty mad at you for not giving Patty Sue the streptokinase shot."

I nodded. Karl leaned forward.

"How'd you get out of that one? I thought you'd never get him off your back."

"The doctors on Abilene told him I had done the right thing. He eased up and actually retracted his first angry letter. Said I was a good son, or something like that."

Karl looked at me curiously.

"You know about his son?" he asked.

"I know they didn't get along. I went to his house and all the family pictures had been taken off the walls. He told me he didn't have a son. So I guessed there was some friction."

"Friction! That's much deeper than just friction, Einstein! That's the end of an oil legacy! They got cattle but they got a bunch of the Eagle Shale and so much oil they don't know what to do with it."

"Did Rutherford have any other children?" I asked.

"Nope. No other kids. Guess he disowned his son or something. I know the son moved to California," Karl said.

"Well, Rutherford wrote a letter of support for me. The immigration guy scared me badly at first, but then told me it was all okay. I had no adverse reports."

"So your green card is on the way?"

"I hope so."

Karl grunted.

"Guess I'll have to put up with you, then. You and your Queen's Royal College of Pain-In-The-Ass Physicians."

"I'll try not to be too obnoxious."

"Good. I got a case for your Lordship, then I'm hauling my hiney down to the big D for my first meeting."

"What's the problem?"

"Seventy-seven-year-old lady, lives out in the sticks, her right foot's hurting. I offered to see her and you know what she said?"

"No."

"That was a rhetorical question, Einstein. Don't they teach you that in London?"

"Why do you ask a pointless question?" I shot back.

Karl smiled.

"Touché. Or as we say in Texas, *touchy*. Her name's Olive Flanders, goes to my church, she's even in my Sunday School group. She told me, Karl, I know you were using drugs. So I don't want to see you. Boom!"

"What did you say?"

"I said, I respect your opinion. I made a big mistake but I went to rehab and I'm totally clean now. We all make mistakes. I'm competent to see you and I'm open about my past. If my past bothers you, then you need to seek medical help elsewhere. No anger in my heart. Just dealing with it."

"I think you said all the right things."

"I reckon she'll come back to me eventually. But you go see her now."

I got up to leave.

"Thanks, man," Karl said, and turned away.

Olive Flanders was a petite woman: five feet tall, slender build, bright blue eyes and short white hair.

"Is this the doctor from London?" she asked Simon.

"The very same," Simon grinned.

Olive held out her hand.

"I grew up near Newcastle. Lovely to meet you!"

She had a firm grip.

"Sorry to bother you. Just got this nagging pain in my right foot. Reckon it might be a touch of old Arthur?" she asked.

"She means arthritis," Simon explained.

"Thank you, Simon. I've heard that before. It's a pleasure to meet you too, Mrs. Flanders," I said.

"I left my husband, Alvin, behind. The animals have to be fed. Always lots to do on a ranch, lots, lots to do!"

I read the admission information.

"So you're seventy-seven, married, an ex-smoker, on medicine for hypertension and you take thyroid supplements."

"Guilty as charged. Actually, I'm feeling rather foolish, charging down here, when there may be nothing wrong with me."

"Tell me what's been happening."

"I got a little hot with poor Karl. I shouldn't have been so unpleasant."

"He's a good doctor," I said. "He's genuine."

"I agree. Maybe I'll use him next time. But for now here's my problem: my whole right foot started hurting at seven a.m. today."

"The whole foot?"

"Yes."

"Do you mean the ankle or the sole or some particular area?"

"No. The whole foot. Everything below the ankle."

"Do the joints hurt? Like on moving or on standing or twisting?" I asked.

"No. Just the whole foot hurt badly, like it was dipped in boiling water."

"Was there redness or swelling?"

"No."

"The left foot is okay?"

"No problem at all."

"Are you hurting anywhere else?"

"No."

"The right foot never hurt before?"

"No."

I was puzzled.

"Let me examine you," I said.

The right foot looked normal. It was cool to the touch, and tender all over below the ankle. The left foot was warm and non-tender. I checked the pulses.

"There's something wrong. I can't feel the dorsalis pedis artery. I can feel the medial tibial."

"What does that mean?"

"There are two big arteries in the foot. The one on the top is the dorsalis pedis. The one in the inner side of the ankle is the medial tibial."

"So what does that mean?"

I paused. I palpated behind the knees for the popliteal arteries.

"I can feel both the popliteal arteries, the arteries behind your knees. But I can't feel the dorsalis pedis artery, the artery that supplies blood to the top of your foot, on the right side. The left-sided arteries are fine," I said.

"So what does that *mean?*" Mrs. Flanders demanded.

"I think you threw a blood clot, an embolus, to the right

foot. That clot has blocked the artery and shut off blood supply to the top of your right foot. That's why that artery isn't pulsating and that's why you're hurting," I explained.

"So what do we have to do to fix it?" Mrs. Flanders asked.

"This is urgent. We have to open up the artery otherwise there will be lack of oxygen to the foot and there could be gangrene."

Mrs. Flanders gagged.

"Gangrene? You must be joking!"

I checked again. No dorsalis pedis on the right. I checked the arteries behind the knee again and at the groin. They were pulsating normally. I checked the left foot. It had strong pulses throughout.

"You're sure about this?"

"Based on your history and my exam, yes. But we need to do an ultrasound to confirm it."

"Let's do it!"

"We don't have ultrasound in this hospital. They have it in Abilene but I don't know if they have the specialists that can dissolve a blood clot or cut it out."

"So what do we do?"

"We need to send you to Dallas."

Olive Flanders was aghast.

"Dallas? Doctor, are you sure about all this? A blood clot, possible gangrene, rushing to Dallas?"

"I'm pretty sure. Just not a hundred percent sure."

"How about just going to Abilene? It's a lot closer."

"If I'm right, then the radiologist will need to snake a small tube into your artery above the blockage and then inject a medicine to dissolve the clot."

Mrs. Flanders considered this.

"If it's something like you say, what's the worst that can

happen?" she asked.

"Gangrene of the toes and maybe the foot."

"Gangrene? Where the foot goes black?"

"Yes. Looks like a mummy. Black, shriveled, dead."

Mrs. Flanders shuddered.

"You scare me, Doctor!" she said.

"Usually ends with amputation," I added, grimly.

Mrs. Flanders groaned.

"Heavens, I don't want an amputation. Dallas it is," she said.

"I'll call Dallas Presbyterian. I'll see if I can get a helicopter."

"A helicopter! No! That's very expensive!"

"Every minute costs you tissue. The delay could cost you your foot."

Mrs. Flanders held up her hand.

"No, no, no. Now wait. Wait! May I call my husband? I need to discuss this with him."

"Of course," I said.

Simon assisted Mrs. Flanders off the stretcher and to the dictation room. She sat down at the desk and called home. I used the phone in the ER to call Dallas.

Minutes later, she hobbled back.

"Alvin's on his way. He wants a second opinion."

"A second opinion? From whom?"

"Dr. Becker. Because you're not really sure."

I was irritated.

"Karl was going to Dallas. He may have left. And I'm *fairly* sure about the diagnosis," I said, sharply.

Simon darted outside. He came back, flushed and breathless.

"Good news! Just caught Dr. Becker in the parking lot. He's on his way to see Mrs. Flanders."

I forced a smile.

"Wonderful," I muttered.

Karl ambled in, sunglasses jammed backwards on his head.

"So what's up, Einstein?" he asked.

"Mrs. Flanders had sudden severe pain in her right foot this morning. I can feel her right femoral and right popliteal pulses but not her right dorsalis pedis. I'm worried about an embolus."

"Whoa! An embolus!" Karl said, impressed.

"That's what I think."

Karl shook his head and sat down next to Mrs. Flanders. He stared at her.

"Mind if I check, Miss Olive? Do I have your permission now?"

Olive Flanders flushed.

"I'm sorry I was mean, Karl."

"I understand."

"You being a druggie and all, I mean, I didn't know."

Karl stiffened.

"Yeah, me being a druggie. But I went to rehab for six months and I've changed. I'm clean."

"I'm sure!" Mrs. Flynn said.

"You don't sound sure," Karl retorted.

"No, I mean it. Everyone at church says you went to rehab. I believe you. I mean, I believe you went to rehab for six months, like you just said."

Karl grimaced.

"Thanks. Let's see now."

He examined her feet carefully. He listened to her heart and palpated her abdomen. He turned to me.

"So where did this embolus come from, Einstein?" Karl asked me.

"She's an ex-smoker. Maybe she's got an abdominal aneurysm." I said

"I didn't feel anything in her abdomen," Karl said.

"Those are hard to feel unless they're big."

Karl nodded.

"Let me talk to you," he said.

We went to the dictation room. He shut the door.

"I don't really know if you're wrong or right. I guess you could be right. But *she's* not convinced."

"I noticed," I said, drily.

"Oh, sarcasm. Very British. Let me teach you something they didn't at the Queens Academy of Wishy-Washy Tight-Ass English Medicine. When you make a diagnosis, you own it!"

We strode back into the ER. Karl laid a hand on Olive's shoulder, knelt, and looked her straight in the eye.

"Olive, my dear, the big artery in your stomach is swollen up. It's called an aneurysm. Blood clotted up inside it and this morning a piece broke off and went into your leg. It jammed the artery above your ankle and cut off the blood supply into your foot."

"Is that why my foot is hurting?"

"Yes, that's exactly why."

Olive looked hard at Karl. He stared back.

"But are you sure?"

Karl looked astonished.

"Am I sure? Of course, I'm sure!" Karl was emphatic. "I am sure! There's no question! I've made the right diagnosis!"

Olive was not convinced. Karl shook her shoulder.

"Olive, I guaran-damn-tee it!" he thundered.

Olive was still suspicious.

"Dr. Mathur wasn't sure."

Karl shrugged.

"I don't care. *I'm* sure," he stated firmly.

Olive looked at him steadily.

"Should I go to Dallas?" she asked.

"No question," Karl said.

Olive gazed at him, then slumped.

"Okay then," she said.

Simon hastily handed her a clipboard with a form.

"This is a transfer form, Mrs. Flanders. Please read it carefully and sign it."

Olive signed it without reading. She placed her hand on Karl's.

"Thank you so much, Karl," she said, her voice calm.

Karl jammed on his sunglasses, gave Olive a hug, and high-fived Simon. He pointed to me.

"Later!" he said.

He sauntered out, whistling.

Olive's demeanor changed. She was relaxed and confident. Alvin burst in and hugged her and thanked me.

"I met Dr. Karl in the parking lot. Thank sweet Jesus he was still here!" he exulted. Olive nodded. To my surprise, so did Simon. I glared at him.

"That really was so, so fortunate that I caught him outside before he left for Dallas," Simon crowed. "Otherwise we wouldn't know *what* to do!"

I had had enough. I decided to save any remaining dignity and leave. As I slunk out, Simon called me back.

"Hey! You forgot to finish the paperwork, Doctor," he said, helpfully.

The helicopter touched down soon afterwards and rushed Olive to Presbyterian. Alvin called later that night. He sounded excited.

"Doc, just wanted to let you know Olive is doing great," he said.

"That's wonderful," I replied. "What did they find?"

"It was just like Dr. Karl said. Blood clot broke loose. Started from an aneurysm swelling in her belly. Clot got stuck in the artery just above her ankle. *Just* like Dr. Karl said. Dang it, he *nailed* it! What a doc!"

I swallowed.

"Thank sweet sweet Jesus he hadn't left for Dallas. That man just saved my bride's life!" Alvin choked with gratitude.

I hung up. My reign was over.

The King was back.

CHAPTER 21

GRAVESIDE SERVICES

"Hey man! You awake?"

"Karl, it's almost eight a.m.," I snapped. "Of course I'm awake!"

"How am I supposed to know when fancy-ass Royal physicians wake up?" Karl said.

I was irritated.

"What's up?"

"Your boyfriend, Simon, just called."

I held my tongue.

"What? You don't like me calling him your boyfriend?"

"Don't be ridiculous."

"Hey, don't get angry. You must be happy, you're his master and he's the slave."

"What do you want, Karl?"

Karl laughed.

"Better than you being the slave, eh? About time the Brits were the slaves."

"I don't see this as masters and slaves. We're a team."

"Yeah, a team. But it's better being the boss, right? Remember, we were slaves of the Brits just like you."

"We were ruled by them. We were not slaves."

"Whatever. We kicked their sorry English asses out and so did you. Is this a history lesson? Let me get to the point."

"The American is the Englishman left to himself," I quoted.

"Yeah, Einstein. Tocqueville."

I was deflated.

"What? Didn't think I knew? Not just another yahoo," Karl

said, triumphantly.

"You still haven't told me what Simon said."

"Your boyfriend said Patty Rutherford hit her head pretty bad. Busted it open. I'm in Dallas. Can you see her and stitch it up?"

"Sure. What happened?"

"Don't know all the details. She was getting ready for her husband's funeral and slipped in her bathroom. Can't speak straight on account of that stroke," Karl said.

I flushed.

"Don't worry, I don't blame you for the stroke. And you did the right thing to not give the streptokinase."

"Is she on warfarin or any anticoagulant now?"

"Yes. Don't stop it, Einstein."

"I wasn't planning to."

"You stop the blood thinners, she could stroke out again."

"I *know* that, Karl."

"So can I leave it in the noble hands of your Imperial Lordship?"

"Yes."

"Make her look pretty for the funeral, okay, Supreme Highness?" Karl said.

"When is the funeral?"

"One p.m."

"Maya and I will be there."

"So will I. I'm one of the pallbearers. I'll hightail it back to Hotspur, no problem. I'm going for the graveside services too. You coming?"

"No, I wasn't invited for graveside services. That's private, family only."

"Family and close friends. Betty and me, we'll be right there. Can you cover me while I'm tied up with them seeing as you're not invited?"

"Yes, sure."

"Thanks, man!"

Karl rang off. Maya smiled at me.

"He really knows how to push your buttons," she said.

Patty Rutherford looked terrible. Her face was covered with dried blood and her right eye was swollen shut. There were several scratches and minor bruises. Simon helped her lie down and cleaned her up.

"You've got a lovely blue dress and jacket," he commented. "Luckily, you didn't get much blood on it."

Patty said nothing.

"I would call that royal blue," Simon continued, as he swabbed her face. He labored to create an atmosphere of normalcy. He kept on talking calmly.

"Do you know why it's called royal blue? No? Because blue paint was the hardest color to make. Blue paint was made from lapis lazuli rocks all the way from Afghanistan, so only the royals or the very rich could afford to have blue color in their clothes or paintings."

Patty didn't move. She looked very sad and distant.

"Also," Simon continued, "this shade of blue was used to create an award-winning dress for Queen Charlotte of England, making it truly a royal blue."

He washed her face again with saline and dried the wounds with gauze. He applied pressure and stopped the bleeding.

"Let's check her vitals," I said.

"Look at this cut over her right eye! It extends down into the eyelid. I daresay it's going to need stitches!" Simon exclaimed.

I looked at it. There was a two-inch diagonal laceration with clean edges. Patty looked at me and grimaced.

"Patty, you've got a nasty laceration. I'm going to apply pressure for a few minutes to reduce the swelling, then I'll stitch it up."

Patty nodded.

"Do you understand?"

She nodded again. She spoke with difficulty, opening and closing her mouth, searching for words.

"Shit. Crap," she finally said.

"Ever since the stroke, that's about all she ever says," Simon explained.

"I know. The stroke damaged the nerve cells that enable speech. Patty only has reflexive speech left."

Patty held back tears.

"I'm going to hold pressure on the wound. Go ahead and check her vitals and finish the paperwork," I said.

Simon strapped on a blood pressure cuff and checked her pulse. He was puzzled. He attached a finger sensor.

"Blood pressure's ninety by fifty and her pulse is forty!" he said.

"Only forty? Are you sure?"

"I checked twice, Dr. Mathur. The oxygen probe confirms her heart rate of forty."

I checked it myself. Simon was right.

"That would explain why she fell. Patty, have you been having any chest pain?"

Patty shook her head.

"Feel short of breath?"

She shook her head again.

"You feel dizzy when you're active?"

She nodded.

"Does the dizziness get better when you sit down or rest?"

She nodded.

"Show me your medications."

Patty pointed to two blue bags with *Ghirardelli Square Chocolates* written in bold black letters. I opened one of them. There was a dark blue urn inside. There was an immediate and angry response.

"Shit! Crap!" Patty howled. She shook her head furiously and waved towards the other bag. I closed the first bag hastily. I took out all the medicines from the second bag and read out the labels. Simon wrote them down carefully.

"Sorry about that. Patty. You're taking a medicine called atenolol, a beta blocker, twenty-five milligrams, once daily. Correct?"

Patty nodded.

"So the atenolol is causing the slow heart rate," Simon said.

"That dose usually isn't enough to cause such severe changes," I said. I reviewed her bottles and held one up.

"This is atenolol. Patty, are you taking anything else for blood pressure control?" I asked.

Patty shrugged.

"Patty, this dose of atenolol usually isn't enough to slow down your heart rate this much. I think you have another heart medicine and the combination is what's causing this slow heart rate."

Patty shook her head helplessly.

"Would you like an EKG?" Simon asked.

"Yes, with a long rhythm strip so we can evaluate the bradycardia, the slow heart rate," I answered.

I examined Patty. Her slow heart rate and right-sided weakness were the main findings other than the facial trauma. I stepped outside while Simon placed the chest leads and obtained the EKG. Simon called me back inside. I studied the recording.

"What do you call two orthopedic surgeons reading an

EKG?" Simon asked, grinning.

"Don't know," I said.

"A double-blind study," Simon chuckled. "Got that from Dr. Becker."

"I guessed. Well, this EKG shows severe bradycardia with an AV block. That tells us it's got to be the medicine, and I bet there's another medicine that she's taking."

"Some blokes have a slow heart rate anyway. How can you tell the difference?" Simon asked.

"True. Athletes have slow heart rates. But in that case both parts of the wave are slow, because the heart is beating normally, it just pumps out so much with each squeeze that it doesn't have to beat often."

"So in those cases both parts of the wave are slow?"

"Exactly. The wave has two parts. The first part, the P wave, comes from the upper chambers and the lower QRS wave comes from the lower chambers. So athletes have few P waves and an equal number of QRS waves that follow right on time. But medications block the connection between the two parts of the heart. So, when you have a heart block, you have lots of upper P waves and much fewer lower QRS waves."

Simon examined the recording.

"I see lots of P waves but much fewer QRS waves."

"Precisely. There are twice as many P waves as QRS complexes, so we call this a two-to-one block."

"That's the kind that's caused by some medicines?" Simon asked.

"Both beta blockers and some older calcium channel blockers cause some blocking. But when taken together the block is severe. Severe enough to make Mrs. Rutherford faint and pitch forwards and dash her head. I bet she's on a calcium channel blocker."

Simon checked her list of medications.

"Actually, she isn't on any calcium channel blockers," he announced.

"None?" I was surprised.

"She is on atenolol twenty-five milligrams daily."

"No, that's too small a dose to cause that much disturbance by itself."

I turned to Patty.

"Patty, are you taking a medicine called diltiazem or verapamil?"

Patty looked confused.

"Simon, call her pharmacy and find out."

"There are three pharmacies in town. How do we know which one?"

"Falcon Pharmacy. It says so on her bottles. Use the dictation line in case you're tied up for awhile."

Simon disappeared into the dictation room and began calling. I addressed Patty.

"Patty, I'm going to stitch up the big cut on your forehead. There's a lot of blood there. I'm going to put some pressure on it for a few minutes first to reduce the swelling. Let's have you lying down all the way. We'll have plenty of time before the funeral."

Patty nodded. She lay down flat. I cleaned her forehead with alcohol and then with iodine. The sharp smell filled the room and stung my eyes.

"This iodine is dark brown. I am doing my best to prevent it spilling on your nice clothes," I explained.

Patty nodded and closed her eyes.

Simon reappeared.

"The regular pharmacist is out for a funeral. The covering pharmacist said that he could not access the records so he couldn't confirm or refute any information, Doctor," Simon spoke with resignation.

"Please give me ten cc of five percent lidocaine with epi and a suture kit. Nylon five-O."

Simon pulled up a side table, adjusted the height, and covered it with a sterile green towel. He pulled on clean gloves and peeled open a suture kit and dropped it on the table.

"The only other people who would know about her exact medicines would be her primary physician and her cardiologist. Her primary physician is Dr. Becker, and he's driving back from Dallas as we speak, so he can't access her medication list."

"Who else would know?" Simon wondered.

"Her cardiologist. She must have a cardiologist," I replied.

"Why?" Simon asked.

"Because she's on warfarin and we don't have a clinic to monitor that here in Hotspur. So she must have a cardiologist in Abilene who monitors it."

"True," Simon agreed.

"So call the clinic in Abilene and ask them if they have a list of her current meds," I ordered.

"Roger!" Simon said, and vanished into the dictation room again. I looked down at Patty.

"Patty, I've cleaned the wound. You're lucky, the edges are clean and there isn't much bleeding. I'm going to inject some lidocaine into the edges to numb it up. It's going to sting and burn," I warned.

Patty stiffened and flinched as I injected lidocaine into the margins.

"I'm using a small twenty-two gauge needle," I explained. "I'm injecting slowly. I'm raising a wheal and then using the edge of that wheal to inject more."

Patty grunted. Simon stuck his head out from the dictation room.

"Doctor Mathur, her cardiologist is out of town, I called

his office and they don't have a list," he announced. "Do we *really* need to be doing this?"

"Is there a cardiologist on call? Can we get the on-call cardiologist's name and number?" I persisted.

"I will try," Simon said.

I pulled open the silk suture packet and clamped the base of the needle with a forceps. I poked the edge with the tip of the needle.

"Do you feel that?" I asked.

Patty looked at me and shook her head.

"I'm stitching up the wound now. I'm starting at the bottom and putting in single stitches, not one long continuous stitch. It takes a little more time, but that way if the nylon snaps, the whole thing won't fall apart," I said.

I started just above her eye and closed the lower end of the laceration. I put another one a quarter inch above and tightened it. A third and fourth followed. I pressed down with gauze and squeezed and swabbed blood and serum.

"I'm reducing the swelling so I can pull the edges together without too much tension. Any pain?"

Patty shook her head.

"I'm going to stitch up the upper half now. I've got four stitches in and you'll probably need another five."

Patty closed her eyes. I stitched the upper half closed.

Simon appeared. He was puzzled.

"Dr. Becker just called. He asked me to address you as Master. Do you know why?"

"Yes. Forget it."

"Is it because the British were removed from India and now you're the doctor and I'm the nurse?"

I hesitated.

"Yes," I admitted.

Patty smiled. Simon was not amused.

"Well, *Master*, I am advised that Dr. Becker, my other *Master*, has concluded his affairs in the borough of Dallas and is in the process of transporting his very considerable personage to its original habitation."

"You mean, he's on his way back?"

"Yes, Master."

"Don't call me that."

"Yes, Master," Simon curtsied and withdrew.

I nodded in return.

"We do this ridiculous routine all the time," I explained to Patty. "Dr. Becker likes to make fun of anything British."

"Shit. Crap," Patty responded, with a wry smile.

I looked at the stitches I had just placed. It looked like a black caterpillar stuck on her forehead.

"Simon, anything about the cardiologist?" I called.

"Dr. Byron Einthoven is on call," Simon replied. "Do you really want them to page him?"

"Yes, I do."

There was a pause.

"They're saying it's Saturday so do you *really* need to talk with him?"

"Yes!"

"They're asking, can it wait till Monday?"

"No!"

"Are you sure?"

I looked up in amazement.

"Their question, not mine, Doctor Mathur," Simon said, apologetically.

"Yes, I am *certain* I want Dr Einthoven paged. I'm certain I want to discuss Patricia Rutherford's medications with him."

"They're asking, what's the specific question?"

"The question is, is she on diltiazem or verapamil along with the atenolol? And if so, then can I stop the atenolol or not?" I said, quite irritated.

There was a pause.

"They're asking again, are you certain it can't wait till Monday?"

I suppressed my anger.

"She's passing out, losing consciousness, cutting her head open and requiring nine stitches on the morning of her husband's funeral. I think her cardiologist could be disturbed for five minutes, even on a Saturday morning!"

Simon coughed.

"I'll take that as a yes, shall I?" he ventured. He looked at my face and retreated.

Patty looked up at me, amused.

"As Karl would say, what part of 'now!' do you not understand?" I snapped.

"Shit," Patty said, sympathetically.

Minutes later I was talking to Dr. Einthoven.

"Thanks for answering, Dr. Einthoven," I began.

"Call me By," he said. "So what's the deal?"

"I'm seeing Patricia Rutherford in the ER," I explained. "She fell at home and had a four inch laceration on her forehead. I just stitched her up. She's got a pulse of around forty-five on the monitor. I think that's why she fainted in the first place."

"Makes sense to me. Hold on, I see it. She's on diltiazem CD, two hundred and forty milligrams. She was supposed to have stopped it. Maybe she just refilled it by mistake."

"That explains the slow heart rate and the fainting. I wanted to stop the diltiazem, if that's okay with you," I said.

"Absolutely. Her husband just died. I bet she's got plenty to worry about, what with her son last month and now this."

I was silent.

"Did you not look after her husband?" Dr. Einthoven asked.

"I'm covering for their regular primary doctor, Dr. Becker," I explained. "I did see her husband and examine him once in his home."

"So you are one of his physicians. Guess I can tell you that I was Old Rutherford's cardiologist as well. You notice his weak eye?"

"Yes. He had diabetic third nerve damage because the nerve was weak but his pupil was reactive."

"Right. Old Rutherford, King of Oil in the big country. Died of a broken heart."

"I thought he died of a heart attack."

"I saw him when Becker sent him up to our ER. The man died of intense grief. Japanese have a word for it, Takotsubo carditis. Being diabetic and having pre-existing heart disease didn't help any."

I wanted to learn more about his son.

"What happened, exactly?" I asked, delicately.

"Had one son. Son and daddy never got along, don't quite know why. Son died last month. Daddy just found out the details and the grief killed him," Dr. Eindthoven said.

I was silent for a minute.

"Do you need to see Patty?" I asked.

"No. Just stop the diltiazem. Keep an eye on her for the next six to eight hours. It's the combination of beta blockers and older calcium channel blockers that's causing this mess. Stop the diltiazem! She should be right as rain after that. Keep her on the warfarin."

He rang off. I returned to the main room.

"You are on diltiazem, Patty. You must have left it at home. Dr. Einthoven wants you to stop it. Give him a call Monday to update him and set up a follow-up appointment."

Patty nodded. I wrote down: *Stop Diltiazem* on a blank prescription. Patty read it and folded it up. She put it in her purse and pulled out a folded gray note. It was thick grey paper inscribed *"In Memoriam, Arthur Marmaduke Rutherford II"* and Patty pointed to the last paragraph: *"Private Graveside Services, McBee Family Cemetery, off FM 2771."*

"Would you like me to come to the graveside services?" I asked, hopefully.

She shook her head vigorously, pointed to the address again, and nodded. I was puzzled.

Simon helped her stand up. She was still attached to the monitoring leads. Her heart rate was in the low fifties.

"Patty, do you feel dizzy? Any chest pain or shortness of breath?" I asked.

She shook her head and gathered her bag of medicines. She picked up the bag with the urn carefully with her left arm. She tried to say something but couldn't.

"Something about the funeral?" I asked.

She shook her head and pointed to the address of the cemetery.

I was confused.

"Do you want to go to the cemetery?"

Patty nodded.

"Now?"

Patty nodded vigorously.

"You can't go. Your heart rate is too slow."

She looked exasperated.

"Shit! Crap!" she said, angrily, and pointed again to the address.

Suddenly, it all made sense.

"Do you want to go to the McBee Cemetery now? Before

the funeral services in church?" I asked.

She clutched her bags closer and nodded.

"Okay, but you can't go by yourself. I'll take you in my car. I can keep checking your pulse. Simon, give me two cc of epinephrine in a five cc syringe with a needle and that way I can give it to her in an emergency. And give me one amp of atropine just in case."

Patty protested and showed me her truck keys but I wouldn't budge. She finally relented. Simon and I finished her paperwork. Patty held up her left hand.

"I'm going to leave that small butterfly needle in your hand for now, Patty. I'm taking a bag of saline and some adrenaline and atropine to inject if your heart rate goes down," I explained. "I want that IV to stay right there."

Patty nodded. She adjusted her two bags and would not let me carry either one. She permitted Simon to carry her purse.

I slipped on my blazer and Simon and I walked her out to the parking lot.

It was a beautiful day, clear and sunny. The crisp, cold air was spiked with the smell of burning mesquite and spent diesel from the ambulances. A paramedic, smoking near the oxygen tank, called out and waved. A light breeze dusted us with caliche as we helped Patty into the front passenger seat of my Corolla. She glanced in the back and noted the dried-out roses and bottle of mouthwash. It didn't bother her. She tossed her bag of medicines onto the back seat and snapped on her seat belt. Simon laid her purse at her feet. Tricia gripped the bag with the urn and stared ahead.

"Will that be all, your Lordship?" Simon inquired.

"Thank you, my good man," I replied.

I drove north on the 83/84 highway towards Abilene. I drove past Horse Thieves Gulch and the Bloody Basin. I took the exit for FM 2771 and the little Corolla bounced and rattled as we wound down the dirt road towards the cemetery.

The McBee cemetery was an open plot ringed by a low barbed-wire fence. Several gravestones loomed amidst the scrub, grainy and gritty, with blurred inscriptions and plugged carvings. Crows and blue jays jousted and strutted, and wiped their beaks on the headstones. A small tent had been set up with two rows of chairs facing an open grave. I drove up to it, airbrushing dust onto a parked truck and a small table with a coffee dispenser and plates of covered food.

I recognized Arnulfo Hernandez. I parked near the tent and Arnulfo opened the door.

"Mrs. Rutherford, good Doctor, good morning! Oh, madam, what happened to your face?" he asked.

"She fell and hit her head. She had a nasty cut so I stitched it up," I said.

"You're the doctor who helped my little girl," Arnulfo recalled, as he helped Patty out of the car. He supported her weak right side.

"Yes. She's the one who had the bug in her ear, I remember. How's she doing?"

"Oh, she's fine."

"What about her brothers?"

Arnulfo's face clouded.

"They got a whipping, like they deserved!" he declared.

"I told you, I didn't think they could have put that bug in her ear. That was just bad luck."

"No, but they put a bunch of bugs in her bed, I know this, and so they needed to be punished. Now they're never going to do that again!" Arnulfo declared.

"Well, I think you may have been too strict with your boys," I said.

That irritated Arnulfo.

"Do *you* have boys?" he asked.

"No. Two little girls."

"Girls are different. Girls listen. Boys don't listen!"

"Sometimes my girls don't listen either," I said.

Arnulfo shook his head. He wagged his finger at me.

"You got to be tough with boys, okay? Boys go bad, Doc. You *got* to be hard on boys!"

Patty stopped. She glared at Arnulfo and jerked her right arm loose. Arnulfo let go and stepped back, surprised. We walked slowly to the edge of the grave.

"I'm going to check your pulse, Patty. Are you feeling okay?" I asked.

Patty nodded. I checked her pulse.

"Sixty-two a minute. That's okay."

Arnulfo and I stepped away. Patty stood still and clutched her bag.

"She's a good lady," Arnulfo said.

"I agree," I said.

"I'm going to get my boys to come clean up these tombstones. Got to keep them busy," Arnulfo said.

I looked at Patty. She was trembling.

"Do you have any tissue?" I asked Arnulfo. "I think she's crying."

Arnulfo looked at Patty.

"I never seen her cry. Never! I forget the Kleenex," he admitted. "Let me check my truck."

"I think I have some in my car," I said.

I found some crushed paper napkins from Bonnie's. I grabbed them and hastened back.

Patty was shaking. Her face was red and swollen and she had closed her eyes. She held the top of a chair for support. Her plastic bag was empty. I resisted the temptation to look inside the grave for the urn.

"Patty, I've got some paper napkins," I said.

She didn't respond. She leaned forward, then straightened up. She twisted her body and turned her head down and looked into the grave.

I put the napkins in my blazer pocket and discovered a piece of paper. *The red roses poem!*

"Shit! Crap!" Patty burst out. She sounded miserable, "Crap! Crap! Crap!"

She straightened up and stared up at the sky. Her face bloated and turned deep red. She squeezed her eyes shut and heaved as if she was about to throw up. I tried to help but she pushed me back. She held onto the back of a chair and steadied herself.

I scurried back to the car and shook the petals off the dried roses. I went back to Patty. She still had her eyes closed.

I read from the paper.

"Oh, my love is like a red, red rose, that's newly sprung in June,

Oh, my love is like the melody, that's sweetly sung in tune"

Patty stopped crying. I continued cautiously.

"So fair art thou, my bonnie lad, so deep in love am I,

And I will love thee still, my dear, Till all the seas go dry."

Patty lifted her hand and stopped me. She pursed her lips tightly and stared at me. She saw the rose petals in my hand and nodded at the grave. I dropped them in. Patty sat down.

Arnulfo appeared.

"You look weak, Mrs. Rutherford. I can take you home," he said.

Patty shook her head and waved us both away. She remained seated, gazing into the grave, so we withdrew. Arnulfo nodded to me.

"Let me show you something," he said.

He led me to a nearby gravestone. It was a rough-hewn cross in limestone, cracked and frayed, burnished with a tempura of bird droppings and red dust.

"Mr. Rutherford's grandfather. He settled here when there were Indians and this land was claimed by Mexico," he said.

"Not much has changed then," I said. "There's still an Indian and a Mexican on his land right now."

Arnulfo grinned and nodded.

"There's Mr. Rutherford's father," he said, and pointed out a more recent granite cross. The inscription said *Rutherford, Returned to the Arms of his Loving Father.*

We looked back. Patty was stumbling back to the car. We hurried back and helped her settle in. Arnulfo adjusted the seat belt.

There was no bag with her. Her face was puffy and she was breathing with difficulty.

I checked her pulse. It was sixty-six per minute.

"Your pulse is okay, but you don't look good, Patty," I said.

Patty choked, coughed, and cleared her throat but said nothing. She pointed to the steering wheel.

"See you soon, Mrs. Rutherford," Arnulfo said.

"Thank you, Arnulfo," I said. Patty waved at him and tried to smile.

I drove out slowly. Patty looked straight ahead rigidly. We drove in silence to the highway. As we turned south, I spoke up.

"I saw your father-in-law's tombstone. It had an interesting inscription. Maybe you could use it again," I said.

Patty looked at me curiously.

"It said, *Rutherford, Returned to the Arms of his Loving Father.*"

Patty looked in front again. For a few seconds there was silence. Then she howled in loud bursts like a tempest; tears streamed down her face, and her body convulsed. She clutched her face with her hands and wept and coughed and sputtered. Slowly, her spasms shortened. She caught her breath and slowed down, and rested her head on the dashboard, still shaking. I looked out the window and forced back my tears. It was hard to breathe.

Karl called me that evening.

"Hey, man, thanks for your help this morning," he said.

"You're welcome," I said.

"Saw you at the church but you were way back there near the door. I was with the family."

"Yes, the church was packed. Maya and I were barely able to get inside the building."

"Then I went for the graveside services and burial. You know, there was something weird."

"What was weird?"

"Someone had thrown a little blue bag and a blue urn in the grave."

I was silent.

"Was that what I think?"

I didn't answer.

"Her son's ashes?"

I paused.

"I don't really know," I said.

"Okay, fine. I think I know what's going on, you don't have to tell me. Anyhow, Patty was pretty good. Held her own. Tough little bird."

"She's a wonderful lady," I agreed.

"Got some other news. Now that you got your green card

sorted out, and now that the hospital finally got some cash from Medicare, they're going to pay us for covering the weekends again. Two thou per weekend. Did I already tell you? Sweet!"

"That's great!"

"I need to catch up. Got three grown boys fixing to go to college. I'm going to make the call schedule. We could just alternate weekends. That work for you, your Highness?"

I paused.

"Would you prefer to work more weekends?" I asked.

"Duh, yeah! That's easy money!"

"Then go ahead. Take two weekends and get a moonlighter to do the third weekend."

"You don't want to cover the ER on weekends?"

"No."

"Not covering *any* weekends?"

"No."

"Why not?"

"I really need to spend time with my family."

"But that's the only time you get paid to cover the ER! The rest of the time you don't get paid!"

"I know."

"You'll still have to come in on weekends to see your patients! Might as well cover the ER, you're coming in anyway," Karl said.

"I need to spend more time with Maya and the girls."

"You sure about this? You don't make a lot of money, Einstein. Kids cost money. You are walking away from a lot of money!"

"Give me a year without call on weekends. Then I can reconsider."

"You're nuts."

"Won't be the stupidest thing I've done."

"You really sure?"

"Yes."

"Don't *sound* sure."

"I do hate to give up the money. But I want to make a change."

"Whatever, man. Tell you what, I'm going to push the Board to get you some used endoscopes so you can set up a gastroenterology center and do some procedures. I'm going to be the primary guy for everyone and you can be the specialist. How's that sound?"

"I would love to start doing endoscopy again."

"You can use the Operating Room, convert it to a GI lab and do upper scopes and colonoscopies."

"That would be great!"

"You're going to be a specialist again!"

"I like that. But take me off the weekend schedule for a year."

Karl laughed.

"Sure. More for me. Your call, man."

He rang off.

Maya stirred.

"You knew I was sitting next to you. I could hear everything," she said.

"I knew," I admitted.

"Thanks for doing that. Your family needs you," she said.

"What about the money?" I asked.

Maya shrugged.

"I was thinking a lot about different families today," I said. "I think I need to spend more time with mine. Spend less time in the hospital."

We heard the girls in the bathroom, as they laughed and squealed and splashed water, and I felt wisps of scented steam caress my face and neck. I inhaled a bouquet of jasmine shampoo and freshly laundered towels. I stepped into the corridor to the bathroom. Priya and Anjali gurgled and giggled and called out to us. I picked up two pink bath towels and turned to look at Maya. She nodded and smiled.

"Welcome home," she said.

THE END

www.ingramcontent.com/pod-product-compliance
Lightning Source LLC
Chambersburg PA
CBHW030430010526
44118CB00011B/569